Obesity

Recent Titles in
Q&A Health Guides

OBESITY

❖

Your Questions Answered

Christine L. B. Selby

Q&A Health Guides

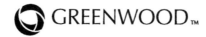 GREENWOOD™

An Imprint of ABC-CLIO, LLC
Santa Barbara, California • Denver, Colorado

Copyright © 2019 by ABC-CLIO, LLC

Library of Congress Cataloging-in-Publication Data

Names: Selby, Christine L. B., author.
Title: Obesity : your questions answered / Christine L.B. Selby.
Description: Santa Barbara, CA : Greenwood, An Imprint of ABC-CLIO, LLC, [2019] |
  Series: Q&A health guides | Includes bibliographical references and index.
Identifiers: LCCN 2018048403 (print) | LCCN 2018049221 (ebook) |
  ISBN 9781440861475 (ebook) | ISBN 9781440861468 (cloth)
Subjects: LCSH: Obesity—Miscellanea. | Body weight—Regulation—Miscellanea. |
  Obesity—Treatment. | Self-care, Health—Popular works.
Classification: LCC RC628 (ebook) | LCC RC628 .S444 2019 (print) |
  DDC 616.3/98—dc23
LC record available at https://lccn.loc.gov/2018048403

ISBN: 978-1-4408-6146-8 (print)
       978-1-4408-6147-5 (ebook)

23 22 21 20 19   1 2 3 4 5

This book is also available as an eBook.

Greenwood
An Imprint of ABC-CLIO, LLC

ABC-CLIO, LLC
147 Castilian Drive
Santa Barbara, California 93117
www.abc-clio.com

This book is printed on acid-free paper ∞

Manufactured in the United States of America

This book is dedicated to all who question whether or not you are working hard enough; you are.

Contents

Series Foreword

All of us have questions about our health. Is this normal? Should I be doing something differently? Whom should I talk to about my concerns? And our modern world is full of answers. Thanks to the Internet, there's a wealth of information at our fingertips, from forums where people can share their personal experiences to *Wikipedia* articles to the full text of medical studies. But finding the right information can be an intimidating and difficult task—some sources are written at too high a level, others have been oversimplified, while still others are heavily biased or simply inaccurate.

Q&A Health Guides address the needs of readers who want accurate, concise answers to their health questions, authored by reputable and objective experts, and written in clear and easy-to-understand language. This series focuses on the topics that matter most to young adult readers, including various aspects of physical and emotional well-being as well as other components of a healthy lifestyle. These guides will also serve as a valuable tool for parents, school counselors, and others who may need to answer teens' health questions.

All books in the series follow the same format to make finding information quick and easy. Each volume begins with an essay on health literacy and why it is so important when it comes to gathering and evaluating health information. Next, the top five myths and misconceptions that surround the topic are dispelled. The heart of each guide is a collection of questions and answers, organized thematically. A selection of five case studies provides real-world examples to illuminate key concepts. Rounding out each volume are a directory of resources, glossary, and index.

It is our hope that the books in this series will not only provide valuable information but will also help guide readers toward a lifetime of healthy decision making.

Acknowledgments

This work was a labor of love in many ways. I know there are others who would have written this book differently than I did. I feel, therefore, privileged to have been given this opportunity to write what I believe to be a series of balanced and accurate answers to questions that many people, including many of my patients, have about their weight and their struggle to understand why they weigh what they do. To that end I am grateful to Maxine Taylor for offering this project to me and for helping me to craft a comprehensive list of questions. She also provided tremendous support, encouragement, and invaluable editorial advice throughout the project.

I am forever indebted to my husband and my two sons. My husband supports me in every way imaginable and encourages me to pursue my passions—one of which is writing. My sons challenge me in ways I never could have imagined and have pushed me to be a better person and mom to them. I am truly fortunate.

Finally, I would like to acknowledge the men and women with whom I work who have struggled with their weight. They have done what so many have done before them and have been left feeling that what they weigh is their fault. Nothing could be further from the truth. Being witness to their tenacity and strength in fighting to find peace with their bodies and to treat their bodies with kindness is an honor.

Introduction

Obesity has been declared an epidemic for many years now, and our country has declared war on obesity. The problem with such a declaration is that it makes the individuals who have bodies classified as obese by a seriously flawed metric (i.e., body mass index) the target of this war. Declaring war on obesity has emboldened many to treat those who are obese with an attitude of prejudice and discrimination. This results in tremendous suffering, both physically and psychologically.

Scientific research is finally catching up with what many have stated for quite some time: what our bodies weigh is not simply a matter of figuring out how many calories we consume and how many we burn but is a result of a complex constellation of factors that include genetics, the degree of food security, the makeup of the bacteria in our gut, and, yes, lifestyle factors that include how much stress we're under and how much sleep we get. Moreover, a growing body of literature has concluded that the diseases linked to obesity do not occur because of obesity but due to a number of symptoms that reflect what is called metabolic syndrome. These symptoms exist in human beings of all shapes and sizes, as do the diseases typically blamed on obesity.

The purpose of this book is to shed light on this research via answers to common questions people have about why and how obesity develops, whether or not it is dangerous to be obese, and what can happen as a result of repeated dieting to try to lose weight. The book begins by addressing several common myths associated with obesity. The question-and-answer portion of the book is divided into the following categories: definitions, causes and risk factors, consequences, treatment options, and social stigma, acceptance, and prevention. The book concludes with several case vignettes designed to illustrate common scenarios associated with those who are obese or who are told they are nearly obese. The book also includes a glossary of terms and a directory of resources.

I hope this book is enlightening and challenges you to think about obesity in ways you had not previously considered.

Guide to Health Literacy

On her 13th birthday, Samantha was diagnosed with type 2 diabetes. She consulted her mom and her aunt, both of whom also have type 2 diabetes, and decided to go with their strategy of managing diabetes by taking insulin. As a result of participating in an after-school program at her middle school that focused on health literacy, she learned that she can help manage the level of glucose in her bloodstream by counting her carbohydrate intake, following a diabetic diet, and exercising regularly. But, what exactly should she do? How does she keep track of her carbohydrate intake? What is a diabetic diet? How long should she exercise and what type of exercise should she do? Samantha is a visual learner, so she turned to her favorite source of media, YouTube, to answer these questions. She found videos from individuals around the world sharing their experiences and tips, doctors (or at least people who have "Dr." in their YouTube channel names), government agencies such as the National Institutes of Health, and even video clips from cat lovers who have cats with diabetes. With guidance from the librarian and the health and science teachers at her school, she assessed the credibility of the information in these videos and even compared their suggestions to some of the print resources that she was able to find at her school library. Now, she knows exactly how to count her carbohydrate level, how to prepare and follow a diabetic diet, and how much (and what) exercise is needed daily. She intends to share her findings with her mom and her aunt, and now she wants to create a chart that summarizes what she has learned that she can share with her doctor.

Samantha's experience is not unique. She represents a shift in our society; an individual no longer views himself or herself as a passive recipient of medical care but as an active mediator of his or her own health. However, in this era when any individual can post his or her opinions and experiences with a particular health condition online with just a few clicks or publish a memoir, it is vital that people know how to assess the credibility of health information. Gone are the days when "publishing" health information required intense vetting. The health information landscape is highly saturated, and people have innumerable sources where they can find information about practically any health topic. The sources (whether print, online, or a person) that an individual consults for health information are crucial because the accuracy and trustworthiness of the information can potentially affect his or her overall health. The ability to find, select, assess, and use health information constitutes a type of literacy—health literacy—that everyone must possess.

THE DEFINITION AND PHASES OF HEALTH LITERACY

One of the most popular definitions for health literacy comes from Ratzan and Parker (2000), who describe health literacy as "the degree to which individuals have the capacity to obtain, process, and understand basic health information and services needed to make appropriate health decisions." Recent research has extrapolated health literacy into health literacy bits, further shedding light on the multiple phases and literacy practices that are embedded within the multifaceted concept of health literacy. Although this research has focused primarily on online health information seeking, these health literacy bits are needed to successfully navigate both print and online sources. There are six phases of health information seeking: (1) Information Need Identification and Question Formulation, (2) Information Search, (3) Information Comprehension, (4) Information Assessment, (5) Information Management, and (6) Information Use.

The first phase is the *information need identification and question formulation phase*. In this phase, one needs to be able to develop and refine a range of questions to frame one's search and understand relevant health terms. In the second phase, *information search*, one has to possess appropriate searching skills, such as using proper keywords and correct spelling in search terms, especially when using search engines and databases. It is also crucial to understand how search engines work (i.e., how search results are derived, what the order of the search results means, how to use the snippets that are provided in the search results list to select websites, and how to determine which listings are ads on a search engine results page). One also has to limit reliance on surface characteristics, such as the design of a website or a book (a website or book that appears to have a lot of information or looks aesthetically pleasant does not necessarily mean it has good information) and language used (a website or book that utilizes jargon, the keywords that one used to conduct the search, or the word "information" does not necessarily indicate it will have good information). The next phase is *information comprehension*, whereby one needs to have the ability to read, comprehend, and recall the information (including textual, numerical, and visual content) one has located from the books and/or online resources.

To assess the credibility of health information (*information assessment* phase), one needs to be able to evaluate information for accuracy, evaluate how current the information is (e.g., when a website was last updated or when a book was published), and evaluate the creators of the source— for example, examine site sponsors or type of sites (.com, .gov, .edu, or .org) or the author of a book (practicing doctor, a celebrity doctor, a patient of a specific disease, etc.) to determine the believability of the person/organization providing the information. Such credibility perceptions tend to become generalized, so they must be frequently reexamined (e.g., the belief that a specific news agency always has credible health information needs continuous vetting). One also needs to evaluate the credibility of the medium (e.g., television, Internet, radio, social media, and book) and evaluate—not just accept without questioning—others' claims regarding the validity of a site, book, or other specific source of information. At this stage, one has to "make sense of information gathered from diverse sources by identifying misconceptions, main and supporting ideas, conflicting information, point of view, and biases" (American Association of School Librarians [AASL], 2009, p. 13) and conclude which sources/information are valid and accurate by using conscious strategies rather than simply using intuitive judgments or "rules of thumb." This phase is the most challenging segment of health information seeking and serves as a determinant of success (or lack thereof) in the information-seeking process. The following section on Sources of Health Information further explains this phase.

The fifth phase is *information management*, whereby one has to organize information that has been gathered in some manner to ensure easy retrieval and use in the future. The last phase is *information use*, in which one will synthesize information found across various resources, draw conclusions, and locate the answer to his or her original question and/or the content that fulfills the information need. This phase also often involves implementation, such as using the information to solve a health problem; make health-related decisions; identify and engage in behaviors that will help a person to avoid health risks; share the health information found with family members and friends who may benefit from it; and advocate more broadly for personal, family, or community health.

THE IMPORTANCE OF HEALTH LITERACY

The conception of health has moved from a passive view (someone is either well or ill) to one that is more active and process based (someone is working toward preventing or managing disease). Hence, the dominant focus has shifted from doctors and treatments to patients and prevention, resulting in the need to strengthen our ability and confidence (as patients and consumers of health care) to look for, assess, understand, manage, share, adapt, and use health-related information. An individual's health literacy level has been found to predict his or her health status better than age, race, educational attainment, employment status, and income level (National Network of Libraries of Medicine, 2013). Greater health literacy also enables individuals to better communicate with health care providers such as doctors, nutritionists, and therapists, as they can pose more relevant, informed, and useful questions to health care providers. Another added advantage of greater health literacy is better information-seeking skills, not only for health but also in other domains, such as completing assignments for school.

SOURCES OF HEALTH INFORMATION: THE GOOD, THE BAD, AND THE IN-BETWEEN

For generations, doctors, nurses, nutritionists, health coaches, and other health professionals have been the trusted sources of health information. Additionally, researchers have found that young adults, when they have health-related questions, typically turn to a family member who has had firsthand experience with a health condition because of their family member's close proximity and because of their past experience with, and trust in, this individual. Expertise should be a core consideration when consulting a person, website, or book for health information. The credentials and background of the person or author and conflicting interests of the author (and his or her organization) must be checked and validated to ensure the likely credibility of the health information they are conveying. While books often have implied credibility because of the peer-review process involved, self-publishing has challenged this credibility, so qualifications of book authors should also be verified. When it comes to health information, currency of the source must also be examined. When examining health information/studies presented, pay attention to the exhaustiveness of research methods utilized to offer recommendations or conclusions. Small and nondiverse sample size is often—but not always—an indication of reduced credibility. Studies that confuse correlation with causation is another potential issue to watch for. Information seekers must also pay attention to the sponsors of the research studies. For example, if a study is sponsored by manufacturers of drug Y and the study recommends that drug Y is the best treatment to manage or cure a disease, this may indicate a lack of objectivity on the part of the researchers.

The Internet is rapidly becoming one of the main sources of health information. Online forums, news agencies, personal blogs, social media sites, pharmacy sites, and celebrity "doctors" are all offering medical and health information targeted to various types of people in regard to all types of diseases and symptoms. There are professional journalists, citizen journalists, hoaxers, and people paid to write fake health news on various sites that may appear to have a legitimate domain name and may even have authors who claim to have professional credentials, such as an MD. All these sites *may* offer useful information or information that appears to be useful and relevant; however, much of the information may be debatable and may fall into gray areas that require readers to discern credibility, reliability, and biases.

While broad recognition and acceptance of certain media, institutions, and people often serve as the most popular determining factors to assess credibility of health information among young people, keep in mind that there are legitimate Internet sites, databases, and books that publish health information and serve as sources of health information for doctors, other health sites, and members of the public. For example, MedlinePlus (https://medlineplus.gov) has trusted sources on over 975 diseases and conditions and presents the information in easy-to-understand language.

The chart here presents factors to consider when assessing credibility of health information. However, keep in mind that these factors function only as a guide and require continuous updating to keep abreast with the changes in the landscape of health information, information sources, and technologies.

The chart can serve as a guide; however, approaching a librarian about how one can go about assessing the credibility of both print and online health information is far more effective than using generic checklist-type

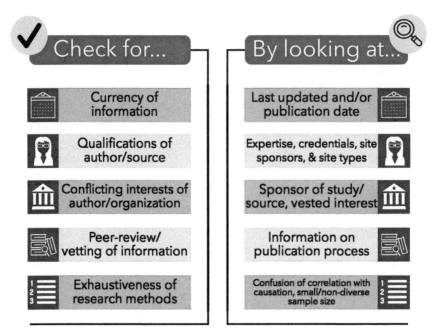

All images from flaticon.com

tools. While librarians are not health experts, they can apply and teach patrons strategies to determine the credibility of health information.

With the prevalence of fake sites and fake resources that appear to be legitimate, it is important to use the following health information assessment tips to verify health information that one has obtained (St. Jean et al., 2015, p. 151):

- **Don't assume you are right**: Even when you feel very sure about an answer, keep in mind that the answer may not be correct, and it is important to conduct (further) searches to validate the information.
- **Don't assume you are wrong**: You may actually have correct information, even if the information you encounter does not match—that is, you may be right and the resources that you have found may contain false information.
- **Take an open approach**: Maintain a critical stance by not including your preexisting beliefs as keywords (or letting them influence your choice of keywords) in a search, as this may influence what it is possible to find out.
- **Verify, verify, and verify**: Information found, especially on the Internet, needs to be validated, no matter how the information appears on

the site (i.e., regardless of the appearance of the site or the quantity of information that is included).

Health literacy comes with experience navigating health information. Professional sources of health information, such as doctors, health care providers, and health databases, are still the best, but one also has the power to search for health information and then verify it by consulting with these trusted sources and by using the health information assessment tips and guide shared previously.

Mega Subramaniam, PhD
Associate Professor, College of Information Studies,
University of Maryland

REFERENCES AND FURTHER READING

American Association of School Librarians (AASL). (2009). *Standards for the 21st-century learner in action.* Chicago, IL: American Association of School Librarians.

Hilligoss, B., and Rieh, S.-Y. (2008). Developing a unifying framework of credibility assessment: Construct, heuristics, and interaction in context. *Information Processing & Management, 44*(4), 1467–1484.

Kuhlthau, C. C. (1988). Developing a model of the library search process: Cognitive and affective aspects. *Reference Quarterly, 28*(2), 232–242.

National Network of Libraries of Medicine (NNLM). (2013). Health literacy. Bethesda, MD: National Network of Libraries of Medicine. Retrieved from nnlm.gov/outreach/consumer/hlthlit.html

Ratzan, S. C., and Parker, R. M. (2000). Introduction. In C. R. Selden, M. Zorn, S. C. Ratzan, and R. M. Parker (Eds.), *National Library of Medicine current bibliographies in medicine: Health literacy.* NLM Pub. No. CBM 2000–1. Bethesda, MD: National Institutes of Health, U.S. Department of Health and Human Services.

St. Jean, B., Taylor, N. G., Kodama, C., and Subramaniam, M. (February 2017). Assessing the health information source perceptions of tweens using card-sorting exercises. *Journal of Information Science.* Retrieved from http://journals.sagepub.com/doi/abs/10.1177/0165551516687728

St. Jean, B., Subramaniam, M., Taylor, N. G., Follman, R., Kodama, C., and Casciotti, D. (2015). The influence of positive hypothesis testing on youths' online health-related information seeking. *New Library World, 116*(3/4), 136–154.

Subramaniam, M., St. Jean, B., Taylor, N. G., Kodama, C., Follman, R., and Casciotti, D. (2015). Bit by bit: Using design-based research to improve the health literacy of adolescents. *JMIR Research Protocols*, 4(2), paper e62. Retrieved from http://www.ncbi.nlm.nih.gov/pmc /articles/PMC4464334/

Valenza, J. (2016, November 26). Truth, truthiness, and triangulation: A news literacy toolkit for a "post-truth" world [Web log]. Retrieved from http://blogs.slj.com/neverendingsearch/2016/11/26/truth-truthiness -triangulation-and-the-librarian-way-a-news-literacy-toolkit-for-a -post-truth-world/

Common Misconceptions about Obesity

1. BEING OBESE AUTOMATICALLY MEANS YOU WILL HAVE HEALTH ISSUES SUCH AS DIABETES AND HEART DISEASE

This myth may be one of the more difficult myths to undo. One reason for this strongly held belief among many people, including healthcare providers, is that obesity has been scientifically linked to numerous, serious health problems that include diabetes and heart disease (see Question 20 for information about diseases linked to obesity). Because medical diseases have been routinely diagnosed among those who are obese, it is easy to conclude that the reason for the medical problems is obesity itself. Perpetuating this myth may also be the fact that the American Medical Association classified obesity as a disease in and of itself in 2013 (see Question 43 for information about whether obesity should be considered a disease). The impetus behind this decision was to help healthcare providers and insurance companies take obesity more seriously, thereby helping to ensure obese individuals would get the treatment they needed. The argument against this classification, however, is the growing volume of evidence suggesting that not all who are obese require treatment. Even as far back as the 1990s, researchers recognized that body size was not enough when considering whether or not someone was healthy. Current research supports this notion, suggesting that it is possible to be overweight or obese and fit, just as it is possible to be thin and unfit.

2. PEOPLE WHO ARE OBESE AUTOMATICALLY HAVE BINGE EATING DISORDER AND VICE VERSA

The principle criterion for diagnosing binge eating disorder (BED) is episodes of binge eating (i.e., eating large quantities of food in a relatively short period of time), which may lead some to assume that all obese people have BED and that anyone diagnosed with BED must be obese (see Question 3 for more information about binge eating disorder). The current edition of the *Diagnostic and Statistical Manual of Mental Disorders* (DSM-5) states that individuals diagnosed with BED can be normal weight, overweight, or obese; however, those who seek treatment for the disorder are more likely to be overweight or obese. The DSM-5 further states that most people who are obese are not recurrently binging and, therefore, do not have BED. Because BED is a psychiatric illness, there are specific treatment protocols for this disorder. Thus, the treatment of BED and its corresponding success rate further differentiate the disorder from obesity. Researchers have found that BED can be successfully treated using specific psychological methods and that the benefits of these forms of treatment seem to last long term. When it comes to obesity, short-term weight loss can be achieved by many people who attempt to do so; however, there are no reliably effective treatments for obesity (as measured by weight loss) that are maintained over the long term (see Questions 27–32 for various forms of treatment for obesity and their effectiveness).

3. IT IS NOT POSSIBLE TO BE OBESE AND LIVE AN ACTIVE LIFE

This myth reflects the idea that obese individuals cannot possibly be physically active because if they were, they would not be obese, and automatically dismisses the possibility that someone may be obese for reasons that have nothing to do with how active they are. The reality is that physical activity can be conducted safely (assuming a physician has cleared one for it) and enjoyed at any body size. Part of the perpetuation of this myth can be found in the visual media. A variety of body shapes and sizes among those featured in the media (i.e., television, movies, magazines, newspapers, and images and stories online) is not terribly common. Although this has changed somewhat in recent years, the predominant body type remains thin for females, and lean and muscular for males. Moreover, rarely do we see an overweight or obese person engaged in physical activity. If they are shown, they are rarely enjoying themselves and are usually exercising as a means of weight loss. When physical activity is discussed by or with someone who is obese, it is usually done so in the context of weight loss. The presumption is that weight loss is necessary (and desired) and that physical activity, therefore, must be done in order to achieve this. What remains missing from these discussions are things like engaging in physical activity for the enjoyment of it and engaging in physical activity to maintain and/or improve one's health, regardless of whether or not weight loss occurs (see Question 9 for more information about lifestyle factors that affect obesity).

4. BARIATRIC WEIGHT-LOSS SURGERY IS THE BEST OPTION FOR PEOPLE WHO ARE OBESE

Bariatric surgery is the formal name for weight-loss surgery. It includes a variety of procedures that can temporarily or irreversibly alter one's gastrointestinal system for the purpose of weight loss (see Questions 31 and 32 for more information about bariatric surgery and its effectiveness). Weight-loss surgery has been practiced by the medical community since the 1960s and is currently performed only on those who have a BMI of 35 or higher. These procedures are predominantly performed on adults and may be recommended for younger patients if more strict criteria are met. Although bariatric surgery can result in dramatic weight loss in many who elect this type of procedure, there are side effects that can range from unpleasant to severe. Any of the bariatric procedures will alter the digestive system, which means that food is not digested in the same way it had been prior to the surgery. This can result in nutrient and vitamin deficiencies, which if not caught quickly can result in nervous system damage. Other side effects can include diarrhea, hernia, ulcers, nausea, gallstones, and death. Even if none of these side effects or outcomes are experienced, the reality is that bariatric surgery does not "cure" obesity. In fact, for some patients, the resultant weight loss is not enough to remove them from the obesity category as measured by BMI. Moreover, the procedures themselves do not prevent weight gain from occurring.

5. PEOPLE WHO ARE OBESE ARE LAZY AND LACK WILLPOWER

Willpower itself is a complex issue; willpower is not unlimited, meaning that we have only so much willpower throughout a day, and if it is depleted for any reason we will not have the energy necessary to do something challenging like changing our eating habits or changing how much physical activity we undertake (see Question 19 for more information about obesity and willpower). Regardless of how much willpower someone does or does not have at any given time, the reality is that there are many factors that contribute to one's body weight, shape, and size (see Questions 9–19 for more information about what may contribute to obesity). Certainly, an individual's behaviors have an effect, but so too do one's environment, social support systems, and genetics. Despite the growing research base indicating that achieving and sustaining a particular body weight is far more complex than previously believed, there are many people, including some healthcare providers, who believe that anyone who tries but is unable to dramatically change their body weight or to sustain significant weight loss is simply not trying hard enough. Additionally, many people who are overweight or obese work hard to try to lose weight and may do so temporarily but then gain the weight back. They may then try another round of dieting, with the same result. This weight loss cycle, which is common for people at any size (see Questions 4 and 12 for more information about yo-yo dieting), can further perpetuate the myth that the individual is not trying hard enough to keep the weight off and is, therefore, lazy despite the effort they are exerting.

QUESTIONS AND ANSWERS

Definitions

1. What is BMI, and how is it measured?

BMI or body mass index is a concept that many readers are likely familiar with. Many medical practices display BMI charts in their exam rooms, and some medical providers may tell you what your BMI is. There are BMI calculators readily available online to quickly compute where your body falls on that scale, and in some school systems children are sent home with BMI report cards that indicate what the child's BMI is, what it means, and what, if anything, should be done about it.

BMI was initially developed in the mid-1800s by Belgian mathematician Dr. Adolphe Quetelet, who was interested in identifying the characteristics of the "average man." His formula was originally known as the Quetelet Index and was not changed to the body mass index until 1972 by Ancel Keys—famous for his "Starvation Study" conducted at the University of Minnesota. As the intended purpose of the index was to understand what was most representative of people in general, it was never intended to be used as a measurement for individuals. Despite this origin, BMI is a widely used measurement to determine an individual's weight status and, thus, to determine whether or not they are obese. Furthermore, given the link between overweight, and obesity in particular, and various health problems, BMI is often used as a proxy for health—meaning that BMI is believed not simply to yield the relationship between your height and your weight but also to be an indication of how healthy you are.

The calculation of BMI is quite simple. It involves dividing one's weight in kilograms by one's height in meters squared. The result is one's BMI, which is then used to determine if one is underweight, normal weight, overweight, or obese (see Question 2 for information about the different BMI classifications). Interestingly, prior to the use of BMI, something called the "ponderal index" was used and was proposed to be scrapped by Ancel Keys because it did not take into account the idea that from one height to the next the body would not look the same. Currently, one of the strongest criticisms of BMI reflects a similar concern. Critics indicate that BMI does not take into account the weight of muscle mass compared to adipose tissue (i.e., fat) or the size of someone's skeletal frame, pointing to the fact that numerous professional athletes are considered to be obese according to BMI despite the fact that they are muscular and lean. Nonetheless, the use of BMI has persisted as a measurement of whether or not someone is obese and as an indicator of one's overall health.

Although obesity may seem like a fairly concrete, easily measured concept, the fact is that the categories used to identify one's weight status using BMI are malleable. In 1998 the National Institutes of Health in the United States approved a change to the BMI categories, which resulted in about 25 million people in the United States categorized as normal weight one day becoming overweight the next. The rationale for making this change was the increasing number of scientific studies linking numerous health problems with higher-than-normal weights.

BMI and how it is used have been met with voracious criticism during the last few years. Critics suggest that indicators of one's health status should include only measures that are known to indicate the presence (or absence) of health concerns (e.g., blood pressure, triglyceride levels, body fat percentage and its location, insulin levels, etc.). Although BMI is still frequently used in healthcare to indicate one's weight status and presumed health status, more and more people are pushing back against this use of BMI as a proxy for one's health and are supporting efforts to use more direct measures of health, including the direct measurement of body fat and where on the body it is located.

2. What are the different BMI classifications, and how many Americans fall into each one?

Both the Centers for Disease Control and Prevention (CDC) and the World Health Organization (WHO) use four BMI categories to classify body size: underweight, normal or healthy weight, overweight, and obese.

An adult, male or female, is considered to be underweight if their BMI is less than 18.5. A normal- or healthy-weight adult is categorized as having a BMI of 18.5 to 24.9. An overweight adult has a BMI of 25 to 29.9, and an adult is considered obese if his or her BMI is 30 or above. Obesity itself can be further divided into three separate categories. Class 1 obesity includes those with a BMI of 30 to less than 35; Class 2 obesity includes a BMI of 35 to less than 40; Class 3 obesity includes a BMI of 40 or higher. Some research has indicated that the subcategories are useful for health-care providers and their patients as the greater one's BMI, the greater the association with serious health problems (see Question 5 for information about metabolic syndrome and Question 20 for diseases linked to obesity). According to the CDC, during the 2013–2014 time period, it was estimated that 70.7 percent of adults were classified as overweight or obese, with 37.9 percent of that number classified with obesity. During the 2011–2012 time period, the CDC estimated that approximately 1.7 percent of adults were classified as underweight.

As noted, these categories are applied to adults. Calculating obesity for children and adolescents can be somewhat different. In the United States, growth charts are used to determine whether or not a child or adolescent is below or above their expected weight. At each checkup a child's measurements are taken and plotted on a growth chart appropriate for their age and sex. Over time, the various data points can be connected to show that particular child's growth curve. The growth charts themselves have predrawn growth curves to help medical providers and parents see if their child is growing as expected. From birth to three years old, the measurements taken are the infant's length (until they can stand on their own) and weight, in addition to head circumference. For children and adolescents, measurements can be plotted on growth charts measuring their stature (height) and weight, and a separate chart for plotting BMI can be used. These charts use percentiles to indicate how the child's or adolescent's measurements compare to those of others of the same sex and age. BMI is recommended by the CDC to be calculated and charted starting at age two.

The categories used to interpret a child's growth on these growth charts include underweight, normal or healthy weight, overweight, or obese—all of which are based on the child's or adolescent's percentile rather than specific BMI. A child or adolescent considered to be underweight would measure below the fifth percentile based on their age when charting BMI. A child or adolescent is in the normal- or healthy-weight category if their BMI falls between the fifth and 85th percentiles. Above the 85th percentile but below the 95th percentile, a child or adolescent is considered to be overweight, and the child would be considered obese if their BMI is equal to or greater than the 95th percentile. During the 2013–2014 time period, the CDC estimated that 9.4 percent of children aged two to five years old were classified as obese; of children aged 6–11 years, 17.4 percent were classified as obese; and of adolescents aged 12–19 years, 20.6 percent were classified as obese. The percentage of children and adolescents aged 2–19 years classified as underweight during the 2013–2014 time period was 3.8 percent. For children and adolescents, the focus of researchers and public health officials seems to be on the extremes in weight (i.e., underweight and obese); thus, there do not seem to be official numbers specifically for the overweight category. BMI is not calculated for infants, but as previously noted, the CDC recommends that BMI can be measured and tracked with children starting as young as two years old.

3. What is binge eating disorder (BED)?

Binge eating disorder (BED) is a disorder characterized by episodes of binging. A binge is defined as eating a large amount of food in a relatively short period of time. Individuals who experience binge eating also feel a loss of control while eating and often feel guilt and/or disgust after a binge. BED was first named and described in 1959 by psychiatrist Albert Stunkard who studied obesity for over five decades in an attempt to understand why some people are obese and others are not, and to determine which individuals engage in binge eating behaviors. Early on in his studies, Dr. Stunkard concluded that fewer people qualified for his definition of binge eating disorder than previously thought. It has taken over five decades for the *Diagnostic and Statistical Manual of Mental Disorders* (DSM) to formally identify BED as a diagnosis separate from other eating disorders.

The term "binge" was first described in the DSM-III published in 1980; however, binge eating was presented as part of bulimia nervosa (an eating disorder involving periods of binging and purging). The DSM-IV, published in 1994, included binge eating disorder in an appendix entitled "Criteria Sets and Axes Provided for Further Study." This meant that binge eating disorder was something clinicians and researchers were beginning to recognize but that more research was needed to determine if it was, in fact, a disorder in its own right or if binge eating behaviors should be considered as part of another existing diagnosis (e.g., bulimia nervosa, depression). Until then, binge eating disorder was identified as something that could be included under the diagnosis "Eating Disorder Not Otherwise Specified" (EDNOS). EDNOS was a diagnosis intended to include those engaged in eating behavior that impaired someone's overall functioning and well-being but that did not meet the criteria for either anorexia nervosa or bulimia nervosa. In the appendix of the DSM-IV, criteria were proposed for use if BED became a separate, diagnosable disorder. The criteria outlined in the DSM-IV were nearly identical to the criteria used in the current version of the DSM.

A binge, according to the most current version of the DSM (DSM-5; published in 2013), is comprised of a combination of eating a large amount of food in a "discrete period of time" that most people would not consume in a similar period of time or in a similar context. Criteria for a binge also include feeling out of control while eating (i.e., the individual feels as if they cannot stop even if they wanted to). Individuals diagnosed with BED experience binges at least once per week for at least three months. Binge eating episodes are accompanied by additional symptoms including eating quickly, feeling physical discomfort due to fullness, eating a lot of food even if they are not hungry, engaging in solitary eating due to embarrassment, or feeling disgusted, depressed, or guilty after eating. Overall, someone experiencing BED undergoes significant distress regarding their behavior and typically reports that they want to stop binging but cannot. Someone with BED may have repeatedly tried various fad diets resulting in initial weight loss only to gain all of the weight back plus additional weight.

The changes made from the proposed criteria presented in the DSM-IV to the official criteria in the DSM-5 involved the frequency of the binges as well as "specifiers" designed to help more clearly indicate the nature of someone's BED diagnosis. The initially proposed frequency of binge eating episodes was at least two days per week for six months, which was changed in the DSM-5 to at least once per week for three months. Practitioners who render mental-health diagnoses are also instructed by the DSM-5 to specify if the disorder is in partial remission or full remission as well as to specify the severity of the disorder by indicating if the patient's symptoms are mild, moderate, severe, or extreme.

4. What is yo-yo dieting?

Yo-yo dieting, also referred to as weight cycling, is defined as repeatedly dieting for the purpose of losing weight. The implication here is that each dieting attempt results in temporary weight loss and subsequent weight gain. Some time after a diet attempt the person will try another diet again— perhaps the same diet or a different one; however, the result is the same.

The person loses weight initially then gains it back. It is common, in fact, for people not only to gain back the weight that was lost but also to gain additional weight, thereby weighing more than they did prior to the start of their first diet. Yo-yo dieting is likely something that seems common to many people as they may either know people who try one diet after another or have done so themselves. In fact, we might even expect those who are invested in weight loss will try one diet after another to find the "perfect" diet and finally lose weight. At best, yo-yo dieting will result in weighing more than we did before we started a weight-loss regimen and, at worst, may result in the development of life-altering, serious medical illnesses.

Research on the phenomenon of gaining more weight than was lost by the diet indicates that engaging in a restrictive diet is interpreted by the brain as something akin to famine. As a result, when food is abundant again (i.e., when the person is no longer dieting), the body will store fat in anticipation of another food shortage. In fact, researchers studying animals have confirmed this and reported that not only do animals gain weight in anticipation of another food shortage, but their bodies seem to store more weight than would seem necessary—thus, they have regained more than was initially lost. Since human bodies, as well as animal bodies, are programmed to survive, and we require food in order to stay alive, we will always experience a strong internal push to eat after a period of restriction (i.e., food shortage); therefore, researchers predict that those who diet will gain more weight than those who never dieted to begin with, and in some studies this pattern has been confirmed. Many people consider the weight loss and weight regain of yo-yo dieting frustrating and annoying; however, the fact of the matter is that over time, yo-yo dieting can be quite harmful to one's overall health.

Scientific studies on the effects of yo-yo dieting have noted that certain types of toxins enter the body through the food we eat and are often stored in fatty tissue. These studies have also noted that when someone engages in yo-yo dieting, certain changes take place with respect to where and in what concentration these toxins are stored. One study found that one type of toxin becomes more concentrated in the brain as weight loss continues. After weight gain, the concentration in the brain decreased but at the next diet became more concentrated again. Additionally, the weight-cycling process was found to result in an increase in a toxin found in the liver. Still other researchers have found in animals that certain cells important for the functioning of our immune system are stored differently in response to weight cycling. They indicate that these changes may explain the presence of some symptoms of metabolic syndrome (see Question 5 for more information about metabolic syndrome), which has been linked to diseases such as diabetes, heart disease, and some forms of cancer. Thus, it is possible that those who engage in yo-yo dieting have put themselves at greater risk of developing metabolic syndrome and its accompanying medical issues compared to those who never dieted.

5. What is metabolic syndrome?

Metabolic syndrome is a phenomenon believed to be associated with obesity and is estimated to be found among 23 percent of all adults, regardless of body size, according to the American Heart Association. Recent research has found that although a greater number of those with metabolic syndrome may be found among people who are obese, it can also be found among those who are overweight, normal weight, or even underweight.

Metabolic syndrome refers to a group of several factors, the more of which any one person has, the greater their individual risk for developing serious medical conditions. There are five factors associated with metabolic syndrome, the presence of at least three of which leads to a diagnosis of this condition. The five factors are a large waistline, high triglycerides, low HDL (good) cholesterol, high blood pressure, and high fasting blood sugar. Having a large waistline is also referred to as abdominal obesity. A greater amount of fat in the abdominal area has been identified as putting someone at greater risk for developing heart disease than carrying excess fat on any other part of the body. Abdominal obesity is also believed to be the factor that is connected to metabolic syndrome more strongly than the other four factors.

The second factor indicating metabolic syndrome is high triglycerides. Triglycerides are a type of fat that are in one's blood and when needed are broken down and used as an energy source. High triglycerides may contribute to the hardening of one's arteries, and excessively high triglycerides can cause pancreatitis, which can ultimately harm the heart, lungs, and kidneys. Related to triglycerides is another type of fatty acid that exists in one's bloodstream and is the third factor indicated in having metabolic syndrome: cholesterol.

Most of us associate high cholesterol with health problems; however, there are two types of cholesterol: high-density lipoprotein (HDL) and low-density lipoprotein (LDL). The HDL type of cholesterol is colloquially known as good cholesterol, and it is important to have higher levels of HDL cholesterol than LDL cholesterol (aka, bad cholesterol). Thus, low levels of HDL cholesterol is a poor health indicator and can contribute to the buildup of fatty plaque in one's arteries.

The fourth factor in metabolic syndrome is high blood pressure, also referred to as hypertension. Although this factor is among those that indicate metabolic syndrome, some scientists have suggested that this one may be associated less strongly with the syndrome than the other four factors.

Finally, the fifth factor in metabolic syndrome involves having a high fasting blood sugar. As many readers will undoubtedly know, one's blood sugar level is an important factor in determining if someone has or is at risk of developing diabetes. The higher one's blood sugar levels, the greater one's risk for developing type 2 diabetes. Glucose, or blood sugar, is typically regulated by the hormone insulin. When working properly, insulin helps the body use glucose for energy. Insulin resistance means that the insulin produced in one's body is not being used to convert glucose into energy and can, therefore, result in higher glucose levels, which results in what is known as high blood sugar.

As noted in the opening paragraph, it is estimated that nearly a quarter of adults have metabolic syndrome. But which adults? Can we tell just by looking at them? Aren't people with metabolic syndrome always obese? Although the metabolic syndrome and BMI picture is not entirely clear, there are studies indicating that those with metabolic syndrome are at greater risk of cardiovascular disease compared to those without the syndrome, regardless of one's BMI. These same researchers noted that those who are overweight and obese who do not have the syndrome are still at greater risk of developing cardiovascular disease. They added, however, that this finding contradicts the previous understanding that metabolic syndrome alone was the primary risk factor in the development of serious medical diseases usually associated with obesity.

Metabolic syndrome does not discriminate based on age, and it is possible for children and adolescents to show signs of the syndrome. One study found that among adolescents in Syria, a BMI of between 23.25 and 24.35 was predictive of metabolic syndrome. This BMI range is in the upper end of the normal-weight range (see Question 2 for information about BMI classifications). Among children and adolescents in the United States, another group of researchers found that metabolic syndrome increased as the level of obesity increased. They reported that among those who were severely obese, metabolic syndrome was present among 50 percent of those studied; however, this means, too, that the other half did not show signs of the syndrome.

Although research results indicate that the risk for metabolic syndrome and its accompanying health problems seems to increase as one's BMI increases, what is not clear is whether or not being obese *without* the syndrome protects someone from developing the diseases associated with the syndrome, like cardiovascular disease. What does seem to be clear is that the presence of multiple factors indicative of metabolic syndrome does put someone at greater risk of developing serious medical conditions such as diabetes, heart disease, stroke, and some types of cancer, regardless of their BMI classification.

6. What are the "thin-ideal" and the "muscular-ideal"?

The "thin-ideal" and the "muscular-ideal" are the current beauty standards for females and males in the United States and much of the industrialized West. The thin-ideal can be described as a female who has a thin body, small waist, and low body fat. The muscular-ideal is found among males who have both a lean and muscular physique. Both body types are typically on display in ad campaigns, on the covers of magazines, and among leading male and female characters in television and film. The seemingly omnipresent and desirable nature of these ideals may lead some children, adolescents, and adults to try to emulate these ideals at whatever cost.

Though it may seem innocent enough to try to achieve either ideal, the reality is that bodies are different with respect to the ease with which they shed body fat and build muscle. For many females, due to their bone structure, it is impossible to achieve the narrow waist of the thin-ideal. Moreover, bodies vary in terms of how much body fat and muscle they need in order to function properly and to be healthy. Attempting to achieve either ideal no matter what it takes can lead some people to become unhealthy at best, and to put their lives at risk at worst. Males and females who do not naturally have a body representing either ideal may engage in dieting behaviors that can lead to yo-yo dieting (see Questions 4 and 12 for more information about yo-yo dieting). In turn, this can result in weighing more than they did before they started dieting to begin with. In some cases, going on and off various diets can also make someone medically unhealthy and put them at risk for serious health problems.

Of course, not all males and females try to achieve their gender-specific ideal. What seems to put someone at greater risk for doggedly pursuing either ideal is something called internalization. Internalization refers to the extent to which someone assimilates or incorporates a belief or idea into who they are and/or what they value. In terms of the current issue, internalization of either the thin-ideal or the muscular-ideal means that someone has decided either consciously or unconsciously that being thin or muscular is very important and that it is worth devoting a significant amount of resources to achieving this goal. For some people, this may result in yo-yo dieting. Others may make an initial attempt at manipulating their body weight, shape, or size, only to abandon the pursuit because it isn't as important to them as they thought it was. For a small subset of those who internalize the thin- or muscular-ideal, trying to achieve the ideal can inadvertently trigger the development of an eating disorder. Research in this area, particularly with the thin-ideal, has identified internalizing the thin-ideal as a risk factor for body-image dissatisfaction and eating-related concerns, which for some people means a diagnosable eating disorder (e.g., anorexia nervosa, bulimia nervosa, or binge eating disorder).

What may help to combat the power the thin-ideal may have on some females includes developing media literacy and self-compassion. Media literacy refers to the ability to think critically about media images and messages. Those with a high degree of media literacy are less likely to simply absorb what they are seeing or hearing, but to question and examine what they are exposed to. Additionally, those who are able to determine how realistic or unrealistic an image is may be less influenced by that image. By contrast, those with less-well-developed media-literacy skills are more likely to be influenced by media messages, and when they are combined with thin-ideal internalization, there is a greater likelihood that such a person would be highly influenced by media messages promoting this ideal. Practically speaking, this may mean that when the message portrayed by the media is that being thin leads to greater levels of happiness and wealth, more friends, and a desirable dating partner, those who are more vulnerable to this message are more likely to pursue the thin-ideal no matter what it takes.

Self-compassion in addition to high media literacy is also viewed as a protective factor against pressures to be thin. Self-compassion refers to the ability to be kind and nonjudgmental to yourself when you feel psychologically threatened. That is, when you make a mistake or someone is critical of you, having self-compassion means you will not harshly criticize or judge yourself, but you will acknowledge that mistakes can be made and that pain and frustrations are a normal part of life. When researchers examined females on their levels of self-compassion, they found that those who had higher levels of this trait were less influenced by pressures to be thin, less likely to internalize the thin-ideal, and less likely to engage in problematic eating behaviors including those associated with eating disorders. For those with high levels of self-compassion, treating themselves kindly included pushing back against unrealistic standards demanding that they change their eating and exercise habits, and that they change their body in order to achieve a particular body ideal.

Although much research has been devoted to understanding the nuances of the thin-ideal for females, the muscular-ideal for males has begun to receive more scientific attention, especially with respect to the negative effects this ideal can have on those whose bodies are not naturally lean and muscular. One study found that over half of the men studied in the United States were not satisfied with how much body fat they had, and in this same study more than 90 percent of male college students wanted to become more muscular. In the Ukraine this number was nearly 70 percent, and in Ghana this number was just shy of 50 percent. Men in this study associated the muscular-ideal with what it means to be a man, which included things like portraying dominance and being more physically attractive to women.

In an effort to achieve this lean, muscular look, some males may diet to lose body fat, but they will also want to put on muscle mass, so they are not necessarily looking to lose weight (a small percentage of males may develop an eating disorder like anorexia nervosa, which can lead to a very thin and ultimately emaciated body). Those who are not able to put on muscle mass easily or fast enough may turn to supplements, protein drinks, stimulants, and steroids to achieve the ideal male look. Using one or more of these methods can have physical and psychological consequences, some of which are temporary and others that may have more long-standing effects. One psychological consequence of pursing the muscular-ideal for some males is the development of a type of body dysmorphic disorder called muscle dysmorphia.

Body dysmorphic disorder involves being preoccupied with a physical imperfection that to others may be barely or not at all visible. The preoccupation with the perceived imperfection typically leads to excessive time devoted to repeatedly checking one's self in the mirror, continuous grooming or skin picking, and repeatedly asking others for reassurance they look okay (i.e., that their flaw is not "that bad" or not at all visible). For those with muscle dysmorphia, the focus is on their own musculature. Typically, someone with this form of body dysmorphic disorder believes that their muscles are not big enough and that they are quite small despite the fact that others will say that their muscles are well developed or big. Sometimes, too, the preoccupation with one's muscles involves muscle symmetry—that the muscles on the right side of the body are equal in size and placement to those on the left side. Similar to those with anorexia nervosa who believe they are fat despite being emaciated, someone with body dysmorphic disorder does not see their body accurately. Ultimately, this preoccupation will affect their life negatively, resulting in problems in their relationships, in work or school, or in other areas of functioning that are important to the individual.

7. What is anti-fat bias?

Anti-fat bias is a type of prejudice aimed at people who have fat bodies. Someone who has this type of bias assumes negative things not only about the person's body but also about what this person is like, such as being lazy, stupid, or unmotivated. Thus, anti-fat bias involves attributing specific personality traits to someone just because they are overweight or obese. Typically, when someone has an anti-fat bias, they are more likely to also have a pro-thin bias—meaning they associate positive attributes with those who are considered thin. Some people with an anti-fat bias have defended public-service campaigns using stigma-related tactics in an effort to address obesity because they believe that being stigmatized will be a motivator for someone to lose weight; however, research to date does not support this contention. Researchers have reported that as stigma-based campaigns have increased, there has not been a corresponding decrease in the number or percentage of individuals who are overweight or obese.

Anti-fat bias, also known as weight-related bias, is somewhat tricky to measure. Will people who have such biases come right out and admit that they do? Measures of "explicit bias" directly ask people if they feel one way or another about people who are overweight or obese. Thus, it is clear to those being asked the questions exactly what they are being asked to admit to. The concern about directly asking people about their biases is that although many people have biases about one group or another, most of us know it is not a good thing and may, therefore, be less likely to admit to having such a bias. Thus, other researchers have attempted to measure people's "implicit bias," tapping into biases at an unconscious level— biases that we have but may not be willing to acknowledge or that we may be unaware of altogether. The thinking is that by trying to measure bias in an indirect way, researchers are more likely to get more honest, accurate assessments of bias.

Researchers out of Harvard University in the late 1990s developed the Implicit Association Test (IAT), which was originally designed to determine whether or not someone who completes the IAT is biased against black people. People who complete the IAT look at images or words on a computer screen, then indicate via a keyboard stroke whether or not what they saw should be categorized with white people or black people based on the rules they were given. The IAT measures reaction time—that is, how long does it take you to categorize what you saw? The founding researchers suggested that slower reactions times when associating positive words like "excellent" or "delightful" with black people indicate a bias against this group. The researchers have since developed similar tests of implicit bias with other races, various religions, and age, gender, and weight groups. The original developers of the IAT and other researchers have concluded that the IAT can determine if an individual may have a bias against a particular group of people and not be aware of it. That is, they would likely say they do not have a particular bias if asked directly via an explicit measure of bias, but the implicit measure would tap into their true degree of bias.

Research in the area of weight-related bias specifically, using what the developers called the Weight IAT, has revealed interesting results. Findings suggest that those in the healthcare field have slower reaction times when trying to associate fat people with words like "fabulous" and "cheerful" and show faster reaction times when associating fat people with words like "selfish" or "gross." The conclusion drawn from results such as these has been that healthcare providers, even those specializing in the treatment of obesity, have an implicit bias against fat people, which can ultimately affect the quality of care that someone who is overweight or obese receives. Even when healthcare providers are educated on the complex interactions of genetics, environment, and personal behaviors that contribute to someone's weight (see Questions 9–19 for more information about what may contribute to obesity), this training did not seem to have an impact on improving the negatively held beliefs about people who are overweight or obese. Despite these results, healthcare providers are believed to have a lower level of anti-fat bias compared to the general population, but the conclusions drawn from these studies indicate that those charged with taking care of people of all shapes and sizes may unconsciously treat overweight and obese patients differently from their thinner counterparts.

Scientists have reported that healthcare providers who have an anti-fat bias are more likely to spend less time with their overweight or obese patients, provide less education about their medical issues, are less likely to provide preventative care or order diagnostic testing since the assumption is that the patient's body size is the cause for whatever ails them, and are more likely to perceive their overweight or obese patients as lazy or not likely to follow through on recommendations. Overweight and obese patients report that going to their doctor's office constitutes a high-stress situation that can lead them not to schedule or keep appointments, and they are, therefore, less likely to get routine healthcare screenings, which may result in some health issues going unidentified and untreated.

Recently, critics have become vocal about the reliability and validity of the IAT, indicating that it does not reveal whether a particular person has a particular bias that they may subsequently act on. They have stated that it is possible the IAT may help to show biases present in large groups of people but not individuals. This certainly calls into question whether or not the IAT is truly measuring bias, and if it is, whether or not what it is measuring has a direct impact on how we behave toward others. Though the measure itself may not be as viable as originally reported by the developers, the concept itself is an interesting one—we may have a bias that we are not fully or at all aware of.

Regardless of how anti-fat bias is measured in others, what is equally if not more important is the degree to which overweight and obese individuals have internalized this bias. Research out of Yale University's Rudd Center for Food Policy and Obesity studied the impact that weight-related bias had on those who internalized negative beliefs about larger bodies. What is unusual about weight-bias internalization is that members of other groups who are routinely stigmatized based on things like race or religion generally do not internalize the negative beliefs about them. Thus, those dealing with weight-related bias are unique in this way. Individuals who had internalized weight-related bias reported that they were more likely to binge eat, which researchers suggested defies the idea that stigma-based efforts are effective in getting people to lose weight.

Being on the receiving end of weight-related stigma, which can also result in discrimination, has been linked to negative psychological and physical effects. Those reporting feeling stigmatized and discriminated against based on their weight were also more likely to be diagnosed with depression, anxiety, or eating disorders and to be dealing with lower self-esteem and higher body dissatisfaction. Physically, there can be changes in blood chemistry resulting in changes in how the body accumulates and stores fat, and changes in the body's tolerance for blood sugar. Some researchers have concluded that although not yet established scientifically, it is possible that rates of cancer, high blood pressure, and other cardiovascular problems may be higher in those dealing with weight stigma and discrimination because that is precisely what is found among those who are dealing with the discrimination associated with racism.

8. What is the fat acceptance movement and Health at Every Size®?

The fat acceptance movement—also known as size acceptance, fat activism, and body acceptance—is generally considered to be a social movement with the purpose of changing how people view fatness and fat bodies in contemporary society. Recently, however, this movement has also caught the attention of legal scholars who have debated whether or not body size should be included in anti-discrimination laws. Related and

inextricably linked to this movement is the Health at Every Size®
approach to body size and well-being, which values engaging in healthy
behaviors as a path to overall health as opposed to monitoring the number
on the scale.

It may seem as if the fat acceptance movement is a relatively new phenomenon given how much social media attention is given to this movement; however, it has actually been around for fifty years. In 1967, several
hundred people gathered in New York to protest anti-fat bias (see Question 7 for more information about anti-fat bias), and two years later the
National Association to Advance Fat Acceptance (NAAFA) was established and is still active to this day. In the 1980s and 1990s, the fat acceptance movement saw greater involvement of people across the United
States and around the world. By the 2000s, and with the advent of the
Internet and subsequent development of online forums, the fat acceptance movement is something that can be considered "mainstream" in the
sense that most people have heard of it, whether or not they agree with
the purpose of the movement.

Critics of the fat acceptance movement routinely suggest that those
involved are promoting unhealthy bodies and unhealthy lifestyles. They
indicate that by saying it is okay to be overweight or obese, the movement
is sending a dangerous message to those who already are or who may
become obese. Fat acceptance activists counter by saying that they are not
promoting an unhealthy lifestyle but that they are trying to educate people about the negative impact that weight-based bias, stigma, and discrimination can have, particularly for women. Fat activists note that
overweight or obese women seem to be targets of those who have anti-fat
beliefs more so than men since the cultural ideal for women's bodies is
explicitly to be thin (see Question 6 for more information about the thin-
ideal and muscular-ideal). As a result, this movement is also strongly
aligned with feminist-based movements.

Within the fat acceptance movement itself, not everyone agrees with
how fat bodies should be talked about or represented. One of the most
significant points of contention is whether or not being fat is a disability.
While some activists balk at the idea that they are disabled simply because
their body size is "too big", others note that categorizing having a fat body
as a disability means that employers and others will be more likely to
accommodate one's body size quickly and respectfully given the laws
related to other disabilities. Another source of discord within this movement is how thin people should be viewed and talked about. There are
those who claim that thin people are a big part of the problem with regard
to anti-fat bias and that they should not be considered allies, whereas

others state that not only can thin people be allies but also that fat people should fight against any stigma thin people receive since no one should be treated badly or unfairly.

Fat activists state that not only do overweight and obese people deal with bias and stigma, they also deal with being discriminated against based solely on their weight. Overweight and obese people have reported receiving worse medical care than their thinner counterparts (see Question 35), have been expected to pay more for their health insurance because of their weight (see Question 24), have been expected to pay more for airline passage on some carriers because they require a larger seat than is provided, have reported that they are often rejected by potential dating partners because of their weight, and have reported losing their jobs or not being promoted due to their body size. Due to these and other reports of discrimination, some activists have suggested that weight-based discrimination should be unlawful and that body size, therefore, should be a protected demographic afforded the same protections from discrimination as already protected demographics such as race, age, sexual orientation, or religion.

Many people have filed lawsuits based on weight discrimination; however, the results have been mixed with respect to the success of the lawsuits. Some people have successfully sued by using the ADA (Americans with Disabilities Act); however, one U.S. Court of Appeals ruled that someone who is overweight or obese can claim disability only if they can prove that they are fat because of reasons beyond their control. To date, the federal government has not included weight in its discrimination laws. Some states and cities, however, have included weight-based discrimination in their laws and statutes. Regardless of the legal issues, one researcher has noted that the focus on body size, particularly as it relates to the health and well-being of the individual, is misplaced.

The Health at Every Size® (HAES®) approach is considered part of the fat acceptance movement and was formally outlined in a book published in 2008 by Linda Bacon entitled *Health at Every Size: The Surprising Truth about Your Weight*. In the book, Dr. Bacon combines her knowledge of nutrition, biology, and psychology to show that what someone weighs is not as simple as "calories in" (i.e., eating) and "calories out" (i.e., physical activity) but, rather, is the result of the complex interaction between one's weight-related genetics, the body's processing of particular foods, the environment in which one lives, works, and eats, the ways foods are grown, manufactured and packaged, cultural views toward and public policy on obesity, and one's history of dieting (see Questions 4 and 12 for more information about yo-yo dieting) and other behaviors. She contends that engaging in healthy behaviors will contribute to one's overall health and well-being regardless of what one weighs.

Dr. Bacon points to the dearth of scientific evidence that dieting to lose weight results in long-term weight loss and improved health as further support for the notion that it is not weight loss that is required for a healthier human being, but engaging in healthy behaviors like eating a wide variety of foods including foods that are known to have health-promoting benefits (e.g., fruits, vegetables, lean meats) but not eliminating foods that one enjoys but that may not be healthy in large quantities (e.g., chips, cookies, ice cream). Furthermore, she notes that physical activity of some kind is important for improving or maintaining one's overall mental and physical well-being but notes that the benefits from physical activity can come from a variety of activities, not just those that most of us consider to be exercise (e.g., jogging, biking, weightlifting). She recommends that those who are interested in being healthy should find and engage in any activities that they enjoy and/or are willing to do. This perspective opens up the concept of physical activity beyond formal, timed, and measured activities to those that can include actively playing with children or grandchildren, going for a walk through the woods or a hike along a river, and so on.

Part of the philosophy behind the HAES® approach is learning to let go of weighing one's self and of the idea that one's weight is an indicator of one's health status. She states that eating healthy foods and engaging in regular exercise is not a guarantee of a certain amount of weight loss, or of any weight loss at all due to factors beyond our control (e.g., genetics, the effects of yo-yo dieting; see Questions 9–19 for more information about factors that may contribute to obesity). She recommends that those taking the HAES® approach learn to take care of their body and to love their body as it is regardless of its change in weight, shape, or size, or lack thereof. Research by Dr. Bacon, her colleagues, and other scientists not associated with Dr. Bacon have provided support for the effectiveness of the HAES® approach. Studies have shown that when compared to traditional dieting approaches, those who participated in the HAES® approach showed lower levels of bad cholesterol, improved blood pressure, and improved energy levels. Additionally, those in the HAES® group found that their self-esteem improved, and they experienced an accompanying decrease in negative body image. By comparison, those who participated in a traditional dieting approach did lose weight and saw improvements in overall health; however, both benefits reportedly did not last. Other research has reported that dropout rates for dieting are high, which can result in yo-yo dieting (see Questions 4 and 12 for more information about yo-yo dieting), whereas those who participated in the HAES® approach were at least as likely if not more likely to stick with their new behaviors and experience an accompanying shift away from negative views about overweight and obese bodies.

As is the case with the fat acceptance movement in general, there are staunch critics of the HAES® approach. Similar to those about the fat acceptance movement, concerns about the HAES® approach center around the idea that it is irresponsible to *not* promote weight loss in some form or fashion as an important element of getting healthy for those who are obese. They point to the myriad health issues and diseases associated with obesity (see Question 20 for more information about the diseases linked to obesity) as evidence that obesity is a guarantee of poor health and/or an early death, and thus anyone purporting to be interested in the health and well-being of the obese must prescribe weight loss. Some researchers add that weight-gain prevention should be part of our health-related efforts because once weight is gained, it is difficult to lose, and over time excess weight will lead to changes in physiological and neurological functioning. Some critics of the HAES® approach have indicated that they agree with the notion that people should not be treated poorly based on their size, and they agree that overly restrictive diets will backfire, but add that there still should be a focus on weight loss for those who are overweight or obese. Overall, critics remain concerned that the message the HAES® approach sends is that people do not need to worry about their weight at all as it relates to their health, a message that, they believe, will encourage people to be unhealthy.

Causes and Risk Factors

9. What lifestyle factors can contribute to obesity?

This is a good, albeit somewhat tricky question to answer. This question was originally "What lifestyle factors can *cause* (italics added) obesity?" The question was changed to more accurately reflect the nature of how body weight is accumulated (or not) and stored (or not). Readers are strongly encouraged to read the responses to the remaining questions in this section to get a full picture of all of the factors that play a role in what someone's body weight, shape, or size is.

The primary reason why answering the question of what may cause obesity is so difficult (hence the change in how this question was worded) is that there is not much known about absolute cause and effect when it comes to how we gain and lose weight and what health issues may or may not occur as a result (see Questions 20–25 for more information about consequences). Lifestyle factors as they relate to body weight, shape, and size typically refer to things such as the food we eat and the exercise we engage in. Oftentimes, the mantra "calories in, calories out" is used to explain how weight is lost and gained. The idea is that the more calories you take in and the fewer calories you burn (i.e., the "out" part of the equation), the more you will weigh. By contrast, the fewer calories you consume and the more calories you burn, the less you will weigh. In fact, most diets utilize this mantra when explaining how the diet will work. Sometimes a diet plan will explicitly state that you must not only eat less but also exercise more, and other times the plan may simply suggest that all you have to do is eat less and you will lose weight.

When considering what lifestyle factors may contribute to obesity, the implication is that these are things over which we have control. In many regards, this is accurate. We usually have control over how much we eat, what we eat, when we eat, and with whom we eat. We also generally have control over how much we exercise, what we do for exercise, when we exercise, and with whom we exercise. There are, of course, exceptions to control over factors such as how much food is available to us and how much food we can afford, what food is available to us and what food we can afford, when food is served to us or made available to us, and whether or not anyone is available to eat with us. Exceptions similar to these are also true of exercise. What we do not have nearly as much control over is what our bodies will do with the food we consume and the exercise we engage in.

Our bodies utilize fuel (i.e., calories via the food we eat) more or less efficiently depending on a number of factors. Some of us have highly efficient metabolisms, which means our bodies use the fuel we give it relatively quickly; whereas others of us have less efficient metabolisms, and our bodies tend not to use the fuel we give it quickly, which means more fuel is likely to be stored as body fat. My guess is that many readers know of someone who can eat anything in nearly any quantity they want and never gain weight. There is a decent chance part of the explanation for this is that the person has an efficient metabolism. We are born with a particular metabolism that can change based on age and the behaviors we engage in. Our metabolism slows as we age, but it can also be affected by the amount of exercise we engage in as well as our history of dieting (see Questions 4 and 12 for more information about yo-yo dieting). Typically, the more one exercises on a regular basis, the more efficient their metabolism will be—but that also presumes the body is fueled enough to support both the body's normal functioning and the addition of exercise. At the peak of his swimming career, Michael Phelps, the most decorated Olympian of all time, reportedly ate over 10,000 calories *per day*. Of course, most of us will never approach the kind of workout and training regimen that an elite Olympian has, but if we engage in exercise at all, our body needs more fuel to keep functioning properly.

Usually when people "go on a diet," it means they are restricting how much food they eat and often what types of food they will eat. Going *on* a diet typically means that one will go *off* a diet, since most of us start a diet plan with the purpose of losing a certain amount of weight. We don't often give thought as to what we will do after we reach that weight goal;

thus, we are usually not thinking about the diet as being a permanent lifestyle change—and if we are, we are usually fooling ourselves since most diets significantly restrict how much and what types of food we eat, which is generally unsustainable. The failure rate of diets in the long term is believed to be over 95 percent. Which means that whatever diet we start, we have less than a 5 percent chance of losing the weight and keeping it off for more than five years. The result for many of us is that we repeatedly go on and off various diets. We start one, lose some weight, but cannot sustain our diet plan, so we stop and gain all of the weight back, often-times with a few additional pounds. We then get frustrated with ourselves for having gained the weight back and either vow to "do it better" this time or to try the latest, "guaranteed" diet plan. The result is highly likely to be the same as the first time, and the cycle continues. Losing weight, gaining weight, losing weight, gaining weight, and so on is referred to as weight cycling or "yo-yo dieting." Having a history of yo-yo dieting can affect one's metabolism and can make someone more susceptible to many of the diseases associated with obesity (see Questions 4 and 12 for more information about weight cycling and yo-yo dieting).

Other lifestyle factors that can affect one's overall health and one's weight include sleep and stress. It is not the case that sleeping more will cause weight loss and sleeping less will cause weight gain; however, sleep deprivation has been linked to a number of processes in the body that affect hunger cues. Research in this area has determined that when people do not get enough sleep on a regular basis, their body's hormone levels change such that they have less of the hormone that tells you when you are satisfied or feel full, and an increase in a hormone that makes you feel hungry. Those who are sleep deprived not only eat more than their well-rested counterparts, they are also likely to eat foods that are much higher in calories (e.g., high-fat foods). Additionally, sleep-deprived individuals exercise less. The amount of sleep any one of us gets is somewhat within our control. Barring other factors, we decide when to go to bed and when to set our alarm. Of course, those with small children and those whose work hours are based on what shift they are assigned have less control over how much sleep they get. There is also some evidence that some people's circadian rhythms are such that they tend to be awake at night and sleepier during the day, which makes working during the day and try-ing to sleep at night challenging at best.

Finally, stress is another factor that is under our control to some degree. There are certainly life events that are experienced as stressful that we do not have control over, such as getting hired or getting fired, the death of a loved one, natural disasters, and so on. Other forms of stress we have more control over and can decide whether or not to allow these experiences into our lives or not. Such experiences include getting married, having children, quitting a job, buying a new car, and so on. As you have noticed, not all of these examples are necessarily "bad" experiences. This means, of course, that whether or not something is stressful is not dependent on whether or not it is bad; rather, it has to do with how much something disrupts your life. The simplest way to think about stress is whether or not something requires you to make a change. You may, for example, love the new smart phone you got, but it may also be stressful for you because you have to learn how this particular phone works, how to access all of the data that was moved (hopefully!) from your old phone to your new phone, and so no. This is a change that requires adaptation. The phone may be a great deal better than your old one, but it may still be stressful to deal with. Of course, this type of stress usually pales in comparison to the stress of a job loss or the death of a loved one. The negative effects of stress tend to have less to do with how many events we experience that required us to make a change—although it is possible to have too much change at one time—than with our ability to handle and manage the change itself.

When under stress, our body responds as if there is a literal threat to it. That is, the body responds the same to giving a speech in front of an auditorium of people as it would to just narrowly missing getting hit by a car. When we are under stress, our bodies release stress hormones, mostly for the purpose of getting our bodies ready to take physical action (i.e., fight or flight). Most stress in developed countries does not involve physical threats to our well-being; rather, our stress usually comes from psychological threats (e.g., feeling embarrassed, worried about meeting a deadline, and so on). Our brains cannot tell the difference between a physical threat and a psychological threat—it prepares the body in the same way. If we are unable to effectively manage the psychological stress we experience and our stress is prolonged, our bodies will accumulate fat, among other things, if the stress hormones released during stressful events are not used by taking physical action for which our brain has prepared our body.

10. What part does genetics play in whether or not someone is obese?

Genetics refers to what we inherit biologically from our ancestors. Thus, in the context of obesity, the issue is the degree to which our genetics affect or even determine what weight, shape, and size our body will be.

There is a strong research base suggesting that the majority of our weight can be explained by our genetics. That is, what you weigh is less a function of your lifestyle choices and more a function of your genetics.

Some of the most convincing research conducted involved individuals with varying degrees of biological connection with one another. On one extreme are identical twins that share 100 percent of their DNA, and on the other extreme are those who are adopted by nonbiologically related parents. If our weight is mostly based on our lifestyle choices, including those that our family members, adopted or not, live by, then we should see, for example, all family members in roughly the same BMI range if they are eating and exercising similarly. Additionally, if we were to task identical twins to eat and exercise very differently, then we should see that their respective body weights would be quite different. The research, however, does not support these assumptions.

Research conducted with those who were adopted by nonbiologically related parents found that the adopted children's weight was more similar to those of their biological parents than their adoptive parents. Similarly, a study that examined the difference in body weight between identical twins who were reared apart found that the twin's respective BMIs were nearly the same, despite having been raised in different environments. The accumulation of research data on genetics and weight has led to the conclusion that if someone wants to explain why they weigh as much as they do, 70 percent or more of that explanation comes from genetics rather than lifestyle choices or other factors.

Linda Bacon, the author of *Health at Every Size: The Surprising Truth about Your Weight*, entitled a section of one of her chapters "Your Genes Determine the Result of the Habits You 'Choose.'" Genetics, she indicates, helps to explain the situation mentioned in the answer to Question 9: how one person can seemingly eat anything they want and not gain a pound, whereas someone else who eats similarly would gain weight. Some studies have examined this by having research volunteers eat high-calorie, high-fat, high-sugar foods and refrain from exercise. They found that there was a great deal of variability in terms of how much weight was gained. Another study examined identical twins and tasked them to eat a diet that was high in fat and low in carbohydrates, followed by a low-fat and high-carb diet. One member of the twins was tasked with exercising more than the other. Their results showed that when there was a change in weight, both members of the twin pairings showed the same variation in weight, regardless of their degree of exercise. When compared with others who were not genetically related, however, there were vast differences in weight change. These findings point to a notion referred to as the body's set-point.

The idea behind your body's set-point is that there is a weight range (believed to be a 10–20–pound range) at which your body functions at its best. If your body falls below the set-point range, it will do what it can to gain the weight back, and if one's weight moves above the set-point, it will do what it needs to in order to move back down. Thus, if your body falls below its set-point, your metabolism may slow down and store excess calories as body fat to get you back within your set-point range. Given that each body has its own optimal set-point range, it is not necessarily fair or reasonable to try to fit your body into what is deemed to be average or "normal" according to the standards on the BMI chart. Additionally, comparing your eating and exercise habits and your body weight, shape, or size to someone else's discounts the tremendous variability in how each of our bodies functions and the degree to which our genetics determine at what weight our body will function at its best.

11. Are there other biological factors that contribute to obesity?

In addition to things such as genetics, metabolism, and set-point (see Question 10 for more information), all of which can affect one's weight, there are other biological factors that have been connected to weight gain and obesity. These include prenatal and perinatal factors, developmental changes that occur in childhood, the possibility of obesity due to a virus, and the composition of one's intestinal bacteria. Prenatal and perinatal factors, changes in adiposity in childhood, and viral infections are all factors that may be connected to obesity; however, the accumulated research in these areas is not as overwhelming as for things such as genetics and the composition of intestinal (gut) bacteria.

Prenatal factors refer to what happens to a developing embryo (the period from approximately two weeks to two months after conception) or fetus (the period from approximately two months to birth) prior to birth. Perinatal factors refer to what happens immediately before and after birth (measured in weeks). Some research has indicated that pregnant mothers who restrict their caloric intake during the first or second trimesters (each trimester indicates a three-month period during pregnancy) are more likely to give birth to children who are at greater risk for developing things such as diabetes, hypertension, and obesity. Relatedly, children of lower birth weights (i.e., babies who weigh less than 5 pounds, 8 ounces at birth) are more likely to have greater fat deposits (i.e., adipose tissue) in their upper body later in life.

Another biological factor that can affect someone's weight is something called "adiposity rebound." Adiposity rebound refers to the period in childhood at which a child reaches their lowest BMI, or most lean state, following a period of rapid increase in BMI (which occurs between ages 9–12 months). The average age for adiposity rebound is between ages five and six years old. Research has indicated that children who experience adiposity rebound at an earlier age may be more likely to be obese later in life. That is, children who reach their lowest BMI in childhood prior to the age of five are more likely to be obese as an adult—this has been found to be the case particularly for females. The research is unclear, however, whether early-age adiposity rebound is a cause of obesity itself or if the rebound is an indicator of other biological processes that predict later obesity, such as advanced physical maturity or consuming high levels of protein.

Obesity as caused by a virus has less empirical support, but some studies have shown a direct connection between certain viruses and obesity in animals. One such virus, the human adenovirus (AD-36), was studied in chickens, mice, and monkeys. These studies showed that animals that contracted AD-36 were shown to have an increase in body fat. Interestingly, however, the increase in body fat as a result of the virus was also associated with lower levels of cholesterol and triglycerides, both of which, at higher levels, are associated with high blood pressure and diabetes.

Finally, an extensive research base exists for the importance of the nature of one's gut bacteria as it relates to obesity. The gut (i.e., the digestive system) is believed to contain over 100 trillion bacterial cells, which are referred to as gut microbiota. The makeup of these trillions of bacteria can affect one's metabolic functioning, or metabolism. As discussed elsewhere (see Question 9 for more information), the efficiency of one's metabolism can affect one's weight. Moreover, one's metabolism can be altered by lifestyle factors including yo-yo dieting (see Questions 4 and 12 for more information about yo-yo dieting), and by the nature of the gut bacteria that reside in one's gut.

Gut microbiota and their establishment in the digestive system begin during prenatal development and involve the transmission of gut microbiota from the mother to the developing child. After birth, things such as how old, or how many weeks along, the child was at birth (i.e., the gestational age of the child), how the child was delivered (i.e., vaginal birth or Caesarean birth), and the form of the child's nutrition (i.e., breast milk or formula), the infant's hygiene, and whether or not they have been exposed to antibiotics affect the constellation of gut microbiota. Between the ages of two and five, the gut microbiota will become similar in composition to what it will be as an adult. The composition of and interaction between the various types of gut microbiota are implicated in effective digestion, the breaking down of nutrients that cannot be digested, and immune system functioning. Changes in the gut-microbiota ecosystem are a part of normal human functioning; however, some changes can mean the benefits of the gut microbiota for the individual can be negatively impacted. Problems arising from negative changes in gut microbiota include inflammation, a metabolic disorder, excess accumulation of fat, and lowered insulin sensitivity.

There is evidence that the body composition of those with whom one lives may impact one's own gut microbiota and weight. In studies conducted with mice, researchers have found that obese mice that cohabitate with lean mice have less of a weight gain compared to obese mice housed with other obese mice. Moreover, the researchers found that the gut microbiota (as evidence by examining the mice's fecal matter) in obese mice living with lean mice had changed and was more comparable to that of the lean mice. Additionally, researchers have conducted what is called a fecal transplantation (i.e., bacteriotherapy), which involves taking fecal matter from one mouse and implanting it into another mouse's gastrointestinal tract. When an obese mouse received a fecal transplant from a lean mouse, the obese mouse developed a lower body weight and amount of adipose tissue.

Fecal transplantation has also been conducted with human beings to treat C. difficile colitis, which can occur when antibiotics destroy beneficial bacteria, resulting in severe inflammation of the colon. When healthy gut microbiota is transplanted in a person's intestinal tract, their own gut microbiota changes and takes on a healthier colonization of bacteria. With respect to obesity, researchers studying human beings found differences in the gut microbiota of lean compared to obese individuals, and also found that the microbiota changed in obese individuals when their diet changed (to lower-fat or lower-carbohydrate foods). Changes in gut microbiota have also been found to reduce the degree of inflammation in the body and to lower one's resistance to insulin. Human research participants who were diagnosed with metabolic syndrome (see Question 5 for more information) and who received a fecal transplant from a lean individual lowered their triglycerides and improved their insulin sensitivity. High triglycerides and increased insulin sensitivity have been implicated in the development of obesity, suggesting that fecal implantation that alters one's gut microbiota may prevent the weight gain that leads to obesity. Additionally, probiotics that change the gut microbiota and prebiotics that stimulate the growth of certain types of gut bacteria have been shown to reduce fat, reduce weight gain, regulate insulin sensitivity, and reduce inflammation.

What is as of yet less clear is how what one eats, how much stress one experiences, how old one is, what drugs or medications one ingests, and one's circadian rhythm may affect the composition of one's gut microbiota.

12. How can repeated dieting impact an individual's weight?

Repeated dieting is often referred to as yo-yo dieting or weight cycling (see also Questions 4 for more information about yo-yo dieting) since the idea is that if you are repeatedly going on and off a diet, your weight is likely fluctuating or cycling through periods of weight loss, weight gain, weight loss, weight gain, and so on.

The most likely outcome of any diet is weight gain, so it would be expected that for those who repeatedly diet, their weight will in fact increase over time. This has been supported by the research. One of the things that is believed to occur because of repeated dieting is that your weight set-point may change in an upward direction. Your weight set-point is the weight range at which your body functions at its best. For example, a weight between 110 and 130 pounds would be the set-point at which some bodies will function at their best, and for others the set-point may be higher or lower. After repeated cycles of dieting, there is a high probability that whatever one's weight set-point was to begin with, it will become higher after yo-yo dieting. The physiological mechanism that explains this is that certain hormones that help to suppress your appetite when you are full are produced in lower quantities, meaning that you are likely to feel hungrier or have more cravings than before repeated dieting. This, in turn, can affect your metabolism, making it less efficient. Other enzymes that regulate fat storage are produced in larger quantities when yo-yo dieting, which means that not only is your body likely to store more fat, but you are also more likely to crave foods that are high in fat. The result of all this is a higher weight set-point and likely a higher weight.

The changes that take place in the body when it endures repeated dieting nearly guarantee that the yo-yo dieter will weigh more when all is said and done. These bodies will be more inclined to store fat and use (i.e., burn) fewer calories because they have experienced too many episodes of "famine" in the form of calorie restriction. Since our bodies are designed to do whatever they can to survive, the body recognizes that periods of not enough food are dangerous and life threatening and, therefore, will change hormone and enzyme levels, the rate of fuel burn (i.e., metabolism), and so on, all in an effort to be sure that the body does not get too thin. This means that when someone with a history of weight cycling eats "normally," they are likely to put on more weight or keep more weight on than if they had not started the cycle of repeated dieting to begin with, thus leading to a weight gain that, on average, is greater for those who have a history yo-yo dieting compared to those who never dieted at all.

Additional changes that can occur as a result of yo-yo dieting include changes to the bacteria that live in your digestive tract (see Question 11 for more information about gut microbiota). These bacteria help to break down the food we eat and can influence how we use the energy that comes from food. Disruption in the makeup of the bacteria in your gut due to changes in eating habits (e.g., eating foods high in fat while not on a diet to foods low in fat or that have no fat while on a diet) can lead not only to serious problems with one's intestines but also to obesity. Even when stopping a diet, it can take a long time for your gut to readjust to the new normal in terms of food intake, and as a result, weight gain may still continue even if you exercise more.

13. How can socioeconomic status affect weight?

Socioeconomic status (SES) refers to the social status or class of someone, which is usually calculated based on one's education, income, and occupation. As noted in the discussions on food availability (see Question 16 for more information about food availability and obesity) and race/ethnicity (see Question 14 for more information about race/ethnicity and obesity), SES is likely a factor in explaining the rates of obesity among specific groups.

The Centers for Disease Control and Prevention (CDC) currently has data from the years 2011 to 2014 on rates of obesity (see Question 2 for information about how obesity is measured) by income and education level. The CDC examined these data based on household income using the percentage of the federal poverty level (FPL). The FPL varies by year and is based on the minimum level of income needed to cover basic needs. Thus, someone with an income that is 100 percent of the FPL is living in poverty as is anyone with an income that is lower than 100 percent of the FPL. People with incomes above 100 percent of the FPL are not living in poverty but may be considered low income, middle income, or high income depending on how far above the FPL their income is. The CDC identifies three levels of income when considering socioeconomic status based on household income: income less than or equal to 130 percent of the FPL, income greater than 130 percent and less than or equal to 350 percent of the FPL, and income that is greater than 350 percent of the FPL.

During the period 2011–2014, the group with the lowest obesity rate, 31.2 percent, was found among the highest income group (those with an income greater than 350 percent of the FPL). Those with the highest rate of obesity, 40.8 percent, were found among those with a household income between 130 percent and 350 percent of the FPL.

When considering socioeconomic status based on education, the CDC identified three groups: high school graduate or less, some college, and college graduate. The lowest rate of obesity, 27.8 percent, was found among college graduates, whereas the highest rate of obesity was nearly identical between those with some college education (40.6 percent) and those who had a high school education or less (40.0 percent).

When considering both of these factors for calculating SES in terms of race and ethnicity, there are disparities based on race or ethnicity and sex that are similar to those reported in the question on race and ethnicity (see Question 14). When considering males and females together, the highest rate of obesity (49.3 percent) in terms of household income was found among non-Hispanic black adults with an income greater than 350 percent of the FPL. When considering household income and sex, the highest rate of obesity (59.4 percent) was found among non-Hispanic black women who had an income between 130 percent and 350 percent of the FPL. Obesity rates based on level of education showed the highest rate overall was found among non-Hispanic black adults with come college education at a rate of 50.5 percent. When considering level of education, race and ethnicity, and sex, the highest rate of obesity was found among non-Hispanic black women who had some college education.

The lowest rates of obesity, by far, were found among non-Hispanic Asian adults. When considering SES based on household income, non-Hispanic Asian adults with an income greater than 350 percent of the FPL had an obesity rate of 10.7 percent. The lowest rate (9.7 percent) was found among non-Hispanic Asian women who had an income of greater than 350 percent of the FPL. In terms of level of education, the lowest rate of 11.1 percent was found among non-Hispanic Asian adults who were college graduates. The lowest obesity rate overall was found among non-Hispanic men who had some college education, at a rate of 10.3 percent.

While the highest and lowest obesity rates are found among non-Hispanic black adults and non-Hispanic Asian adults, respectively, these rates are not purely a function of not being educated enough or earning enough money. If that were the case, we'd see the highest obesity rates among those with the least amount of education and the lowest income levels. Thus, while these data show which groups are more likely to be obese than others, these data also contribute to the murkiness of trying to pinpoint specific causes of obesity.

14. How does race/ethnicity affect weight?

The question of how race and ethnicity affect weight is not quite as simple as it might seem. Knowing that one or more racial or ethnic groups may be more prone to obesity than another implies that race and ethnicity might be a cause of obesity. The reality is that race and ethnicity likely interact with other factors such as food availability (see Question 16 for more information about food availability and obesity), socioeconomic status (see Question 13 for more information about socioeconomic status and obesity), and a sedentary lifestyle (see Question 9 for more information about lifestyle factors and obesity). In fact, one study entitled *Adolescents' Health Behaviors and Obesity: Does Race Affect This Epidemic?* identified what the authors called "causal pathways" that outlined what factors are involved prior to someone's becoming obese. The study identified factors such as vigorous physical activity, sedentary activity, socioeconomic status, and hours of sleep as affecting one's obesity status. Although the pathways were different between Caucasian and black participants, the results of the study only suggest that different circumstances and behaviors affect each group but are not necessarily the true cause. In the following paragraphs, what will be presented is a brief discussion of which racial and ethnic groups are more likely to have members who are obese compared to others, with the understanding that race and ethnicity are not necessarily the cause of obesity in these groups.

As noted in Question 15, on age and weight, adults over the age of 20 are more likely to be obese compared to younger age groups. Overall, the rate of obesity among adults was calculated by the Centers for Disease Control and Prevention (CDC) to be just shy of 40 percent in 2015–2016, with the highest rate found among those between the ages of 40 and 59 at 42.8 percent. According to the CDC, the rate of adult obesity among different racial and ethnic groups varies widely, with the lowest rate found among non-Hispanic Asian adults at 12.7 percent. The highest rates were found to be 47 percent and 46.8 percent among Hispanic adults and non-Hispanic black adults, respectively. Non-Hispanic white adults were reported to have an obesity rate of 37.9 percent. In all racial and ethnic categories, women were reported to have higher rates of obesity than men, with the highest obesity rate overall found among non-Hispanic black women at 54.8 percent.

Obesity rates can be calculated as young as age two and can also be examined by race and ethnic background. Thus, the data on obesity rates among youth span ages 2–19. According to the CDC, the overall rate of obesity among the youth population of the United States between 2015 and 2016 was 18.5 percent, with the highest rate found among those aged 12–19 years. Examining these data by race and ethnicity reveals a nearly identical picture as that found among adults. The lowest rates of obesity were found among non-Hispanic Asian youth (11 percent) followed by non-Hispanic white youth (14.1 percent). The highest rates of obesity were found among non-Hispanic black youth (22 percent) and Hispanic youth (25.8 percent). Differing from that found among adults, the highest rate of obesity when broken down by sex was found among Hispanic boys (28 percent). Additionally, boys had higher rates of obesity among other racial and ethnic groups except among non-Hispanic black youth. In this group, girls had a rate of 25.1 percent compared to the boys at 19 percent.

15. How does age affect weight?

Most readers likely know that although obesity rates among human beings in general are a concern for most developed countries and most obesity prevention-efforts focus on children, the fact is that the highest rates of obesity are found among adults 20 years and older. Obesity rates steadily increase with age until older adulthood. Thirty-two percent of young adults aged 20–39 years old are classified as obese, whereas those aged 40–49 years have the highest rate of obesity at just over 40 percent. Adults over the age of 60 have a somewhat lower obesity rate at around 37 percent; however, this may be explained by an increase in disease processes, which can result in weight loss.

There are a number of factors that may affect one's weight as we age. One factor involves an individual's metabolism. An efficient or "fast" metabolism means that one's body burns fuel (i.e., calories) relatively quickly, thus not allowing for much if any fat storage. Regardless of how efficient one's metabolism is, it will begin to slow down when we reach our 20s, meaning that our bodies will naturally burn fewer calories each day. A factor that does affect this is the transition from muscle tissue to fat in those who are not active or as active as they had been when they were younger. Since pound for pound muscle burns more energy than fat, the more muscle you have, the more energy your body will use. Thus, although

our metabolisms predictably slow down with age, the most important factor is the degree to which we remain active.

Other changes that occur in the body as we age include the type and
location of fat our bodies store. For example, fat just below the skin,
referred to as subcutaneous fat, decreases with age; however, fat stored in
the abdominal area, referred to as visceral fat, increases with age. Visceral
fat is a factor in metabolic syndrome, which is associated with a number
of serious medical conditions including heart disease, stroke, and early
death (see Question 5 for more information about metabolic syndrome).

The combination of decreased muscle mass and increased abdominal
fat also affects how sensitive your body is to insulin. Insulin helps the body
regulate how much sugar, in the form of glucose, is in your blood. As we
age and our body composition changes, our bodies also become less sensitive to insulin, also referred to as being insulin resistant. When the body
is insulin resistant, more insulin is needed to keep one's blood sugar levels
within healthy limits. If one's body cannot keep up, insulin injections may
be required. Without managing insulin resistance, problems such as high
blood pressure and higher cholesterol levels can occur.

Despite the slowing down of one's metabolism, weight gain is not inevitable. Again, it boils down to understanding how your body is changing
and how you treat your body. Continuing to exercise or starting an exercise routine (assuming you are medically cleared to engage in exercise)
along with eating reasonable types and amounts of food can help to keep
one's weight stable. As many adults know when they are well above their
20s, they cannot keep doing what they were doing when they were
younger and expect to stay at the same weight or even to feel as healthy
as they once did. The most important factor, however, is maintaining
one's muscle mass. Muscle mass declines as we age, and this is referred to
as sarcopenia. Therefore, it is important not only for one's weight but
one's overall health to continue or begin an exercise routine.

Thinner is not, however, necessarily better as you age. Recent research
has confirmed the notion that a slightly higher body weight (i.e., overweight
or low-level obesity) is associated with greater longevity compared to those
who are normal weight or underweight or those with a very high BMI.

16. How does food availability affect weight?

In the worlds of research and governmental programming, the availability
of food or lack thereof is referred to as food security. The degree of food
security is often identified by region or area of a state. A food insecure

region of the United States is defined as not having dependable access to enough food that is both affordable and nutritious. There are some regions in the United States that are considered food deserts. Those who live in food deserts will have difficulty finding and being able to afford nutritious food (e.g., fresh fruits and vegetables). As many as 29 million people in the United States are believed to live in food deserts, which means there is not a supermarket or farm stand within one mile of a household in an urban area or within 10 miles of a household in a rural area. Moreover, someone living in a food desert may or may not have a reliable form of transportation to get to a store or farm stand. The idea here is not that there is necessarily a shortage of food altogether (although that certainly occurs); rather, that there is a shortage of affordable, healthy foods. Thus, without access to affordable, nutritious food, residents in food deserts or who are in food insecure areas may rely entirely or often on quick, cheap, convenience types of food, which are often considered "junk food" or at the very least not terribly healthy.

In the United States, by far, most of the food insecure areas are in the South, accounting for 90 percent of food insecure regions. Half of food insecure areas are found in rural regions, and just over 25 percent are found in metropolitan areas. Some of the factors that affect which regions and ultimately which households are food insecure include things such as household income and employment status, the number of children living in single- or dual-parent households, average wages in the state itself, cost of housing, and degree of participation in programs designed to help people access food. Food insecurity also affects different racial and ethnic populations disproportionately. In black and Latino groups, approximately 25 percent of families are food insecure compared to 11 percent of non-Latino whites. When the majority of a region is populated by those who are Native American or Alaskan Native, food insecurity rates can be 40 percent or higher. These areas and populations also tend to see a higher rate of obesity compared to other regions of the country or racial and ethnic groups.

There is a significant connection between being food insecure and obesity. On the surface, without understanding what food insecurity really means, this can seem counterintuitive. If someone cannot count on having access to food, shouldn't they be below what would be considered a normal weight? Of course, knowing that it is not so much that there is little or no food when considering food insecurity but, rather, access to affordable, healthy food, the connection can make more sense. One researcher attempted to make sense of how and why food insecurity is associated with obesity. The two possible explanations are that food insecurity and obesity are connected as a result of consuming appealing and calorically dense foods, or that the two factors are connected due to lack of knowledge, time, and resources needed to eat healthier and engage in regular physical activity. Other researchers have noted that the connection between food insecurity and obesity "is expected given that both are consequences of economic and social disadvantage." Thus, as other researchers have concluded, it is not necessarily the case that being food insecure causes obesity but that a combination of lack of access to healthy foods, eating larger portions of food (often associated with less healthy foods), and living a more sedentary lifestyle in part due to challenges associated with engaging in healthy behaviors—all of which are associated with being economically disadvantaged—seems to explain the connection between food insecurity and obesity.

When food insecurity or living in a food desert leads to skipping meals or not eating enough so that others in the household can have more food (e.g., children, dependent older adults), such individuals may eat voraciously when food is more abundant. As discussed in the context of yo-yo dieting or weight cycling (see Questions 4 and 12 for more information), patterns of caloric restriction (in this case not due to a diet but due to the lack of food) and overeating can lead not only to eating behaviors that can reflect an eating disorder but also to metabolic changes that make fat storage and weight gain predictable. Additionally, stress levels tend to be high among those who live in low-income households. Too much stress over time leads to consistent release of stress hormones and changes in metabolic functioning, which are also associated with weight gain and obesity (see Question 9 for more information about lifestyle factors associated with obesity).

17. What role do medications play in an individual's weight?

There are a number of medications that can contribute to weight gain. Depending on the purpose of taking the medication and the availability of alternative medications, it may be possible to change medication to one that does not have weight gain as a side effect. Stopping a current medication, however, is never recommended until your prescribing provider is consulted.

There can be a variety of reasons why you have noticed weight gain associated with a particular medication. Sometimes the medication itself will cause weight gain, whereas for other medications, weight gain may occur because of a side effect such as appetite stimulation, which can result in your eating more than you normally would. Other medications may interact with other processes in your body, resulting in weight gain. These may include medications that affect how your body metabolizes and stores blood sugar (i.e., glucose), resulting in greater fat storage, often in your abdominal area. Other medications may affect your metabolism by slowing it down, thereby resulting in fewer calories burned. Finally, some medications may cause your body to retain fluid, which adds weight, but not fat, to your body, and other medications may result in feeling fatigued or having shortness of breath, which may alter your normal exercise routine, resulting in less exercise overall. How much weight a particular person gains because of a medication will vary. Some may gain a significant amount of weight over the course of a year, whereas others may notice a similar weight gain in a matter of months.

The types of medications that can result in weight gain are usually identified by the class or category of medication, though not necessarily all of the medications in a particular class will have weight gain as a side effect. The most common classes of medications that are known to cause weight gain are antidepressants and mood stabilizers, antipsychotics, anti-seizure medications, steroids, beta blockers, medications for the treatment of allergies, and medications for the treatment of diabetes. In the following paragraphs, a brief description and list of medications by common name will be presented. It is possible that any prescription medication you have that falls into one of the categories may be known to you by its trade name (e.g., Zoloft®). A quick call to your prescribing provider or pharmacist or an Internet search can tell you what the common name is for your medication (e.g., sertraline).

Antidepressant medications include many subclasses or different types of antidepressants. In terms of weight gain, the subclasses of antidepressant medications that have this potential side effect include tricyclic antidepressants and selective serotonin reuptake inhibitors (SSRIs). Tricyclics include amitriptyline, doxepin, imipramine, nortriptyline, trimipramine, and mirtazapine. SSRIs with weight gain as a possible side effect include sertraline, paroxetine, and fluvoxamine. These medications can affect your mood by making you feel better overall but can also interfere with your appetite and how your body metabolizes the food you consume. Mood-stabilizing medications help to control the lows of depression and the highs of mania for those with bipolar disorder. Mood-stabilizing medications known to cause weight gain include clozapine, lithium, olanzapine, quetiapine, and risperidone (note: some of these are also classified as antipsychotic medications). These medications have a similar effect as antidepressants—they can affect one's metabolism and appetite.

Antipsychotic medications are often used to treat the symptoms of schizophrenia but are also prescribed for those with bipolar disorder or severe anxiety or depression. Antipsychotic medications associated with weight gain include haloperidol, loxapine, clozapine, chlorpromazine, fluphenazine, risperidone, olanzapine, and quetiapine. These antipsychotics are believed to result in weight gain due to an increase in appetite.

Antiseizure or anticonvulsant medications used to treat seizure disorders are also sometimes used to treat migraines. Those associated with weight gain include valproic acid, carbamazepine, and gabapentin. Sometimes the tricyclic antidepressant amitriptyline may be prescribed to treat symptoms associated with this class of medication. Antiseizure medications can make it more difficult for you to recognize when you are full. You may also experience an increase in your appetite combined with a slower metabolism and fluid retention. Some research demonstrated that in some cases there was a specific craving for "fast food."

Steroids, also referred to as corticosteroids, can be prescribed to treat inflammatory diseases, asthma, symptoms associated with menopause, and to prevent pregnancy (i.e., birth control). Medications in this class include prednisone, cortisone, budesonide, ciclesonide, fluticasone, estrogen, and progestogens. It is important to note that this class of steroids does not cause you to "bulk up" like a bodybuilder. Those steroids are different from corticosteroids. Corticosteroids affect your metabolism, and taking these medications, long term, can result in an increased appetite as well as greater fat storage in the abdomen.

Beta blockers are used to treat problems with heart functioning. Those that can cause weight gain include acebutolol, atenolol, metoprolol, and propranolol. The treating effects of these medications—slowing your heart rate and lowering your blood pressure—can mean that you don't burn as many calories even when exercising. Additionally, some people experience fatigue when taking these medications—which can, of course, mean you are less likely to exercise.

Allergy medications, also known as antihistamines, associated with weight gain include cetirizine, diphenhydramine, fexofenadine, and loratadine. These medications do not require a prescription and function by blocking histamines, which are the culprit in many allergy symptoms. By blocking histamines from doing what they normally do, a consequence can be weight gain. It is unclear what mechanism takes place to promote weight gain; however, one hypothesis is that antihistamines may increase one's appetite. Additionally, some people experience drowsiness when taking antihistamines, which can affect your desire to engage in exercise.

Finally, medications for the purpose of treating diabetes that are also associated with weight gain are insulins including insulin lispro, insulin aspart, and insulin glulisine; thiazolidinediones (TZDs) including pioglitazone; sulfonylureas (SUs) such as chlorpropamide, tolbutamide, glimepriride, glipizide, glyburide; and meglitinides such as nateglinide and repaglinide. These medications affect blood sugar levels. Some medications may result in initial weight gain until your body gets used to how the medication works, whereas other medications may treat nearly all calories consumed as fuel to be stored as fat.

The medications listed in the previous paragraphs are not an exhaustive list. New medications are developed frequently, and some are no longer prescribed or are "taken off the market." Thus, it is always recommended that those taking any medications (or supplements, regardless of whether they are prescribed or purchased over the counter) ask as many questions as possible when taking or prior to taking a new medication. Knowing what side effects may be possible with a particular medication and what side effects you do not want to have will allow you to work more effectively with your prescriber, which will further result in a medication that effectively addresses your symptoms while not resulting in unwanted side effects. Sometimes, however, in order to treat a particular issue, whether medical or psychological, there may not be an alternative medication, or the alternatives do not adequately address your symptoms. Then the conversation you may have with your provider revolves around managing the side effects or determining if the side effects are worse than continuing to experience the symptoms associated with the issue. It is not, however, ever recommended to discontinue any prescription medication without first consulting with your prescribing provider.

18. What medical conditions might affect someone's weight?

As implied by the title of this section (Causes and Risk Factors), there can be myriad reasons why someone may gain weight or have a body that is classified as obese. In addition to genetics, biological factors, lifestyle factors, economic issues, and some medications (see Questions 9–17 for information about other causes), it is possible that the reason for someone's weight gain has to do with a medical problem that may or may not have been diagnosed.

The thyroid gland in your body is pivotal in regulating your body's metabolism. When functioning properly, the thyroid releases the optimal amount of thyroid hormones to ensure your body is not burning too much or too little energy in the form of calories. With an underactive thyroid, or hypothyroidism, not enough thyroid hormone is produced, resulting in a slower metabolism, which is often accompanied by weight gain.

Cushing's syndrome is a rare medical condition and occurs due to an abnormally high level of cortisol. Cortisol influences myriad processes in the body including helping to regulate blood sugar, to regulate your metabolism, to reduce inflammation, to form memories, to regulate the balance of salt and water in your body, and to regulate blood pressure. Cushing's syndrome can develop as a result of long-term corticosteroid use and is also known as iatrogenic Cushing's syndrome. It can also develop as a consequence of a tumor, and if so is referred to as endogenous Cushing's syndrome. Weight gain associated with either form of Cushing's syndrome usually occurs in the chest, face, and stomach due to fat directly distributed to these areas.

PCOS or polycystic ovary syndrome is a fairly common medical issue affecting women and how their ovaries function. PCOS is believed to be the result of problems with hormone levels such as insulin and androgens (e.g., testosterone). Symptoms accompanying PCOS include irregular menstrual cycles, including no periods or heavy periods, pain in the pelvic area, extra hair (often on the face), acne, patches of dark skin, and weight gain. The weight gain associated with PCOS typically occurs in the abdominal area, which is usually where men accumulate body fat (women tend to accumulate more body fat in the hips and thighs, resulting in a "pear" shape). Thus, the weight gain associated with PCOS is believed to be due to increased levels of male hormones (androgens).

Major depressive disorder (i.e., depression) can be accompanied by weight gain. There are a number of symptoms associated with the diagnosis of depression, which include weight loss or weight gain. Either is usually associated with one's appetite. Some people with depression have no appetite, whereas others have an increased appetite. Food may be used by some as a coping mechanism for low mood, which means they will eat when they do not feel good. This can often result in overeating and weight gain, which in turn can make someone feel worse about themselves, resulting in continued overeating due to feeling bad.

Other issues that are not necessarily medical conditions but that can result in weight gain include sleep deprivation, stress, or change in work schedule, which is often associated with disrupted sleep.

19. Do obese people lack willpower?

Willpower is an often-used term to describe the effort used to engage in a particular behavior or the effort used to resist engaging in a particular behavior. Other terms for willpower are self-control and self-discipline. Many people believe that self-control or willpower is essentially unlimited. If you've got willpower to do or avoid doing one thing, then you should have it to do or avoid doing another thing. What such a perspective fails to take into consideration is the amount of energy required to exert this kind of self-control and the possibility of what some researchers call willpower depletion.

Willpower can be thought of in terms of delaying gratification—that is, you resist what you want in the short term in order to benefit in the long term, the implication being that not resisting what you want in the short term will impede your ability to get what you want in the long term. One example: researchers have found that the best predictor of academic success is not how smart you are (i.e., your IQ score) but your degree of self-discipline. Can you routinely resist going out with friends when you have a lot of homework to do or you have to study for an exam? If so, then you have high self-discipline or high self-control. Another example that is not only relevant to this book but is also familiar to most people is that having a long-term goal of losing weight means that one has to repeatedly resist short-term desires such as eating high-fat, high-calorie foods on a regular basis, particularly when under significant stress. If we are able to do so, then we are believed to have high self-control or strong willpower.

So what happens when we are unable to resist short-term desires in order to meet our longer-term goals? Does that mean we don't have willpower or self-discipline at all? Does that mean we are weak and there is something wrong with us? The answer to both questions is no.

There is some evidence pointing to specific brain patterns that differentiate those with high self-control and those who struggle to control their impulses. The primary region of the brain indicated in self-control is called the prefrontal cortex. This part of the brain (located behind your forehead) is involved with what are called executive functioning skills. These skills, when well developed, allow us to understand right from wrong, make choices, consider consequences when making choices, and, of course, delay gratification for a longer-term goal. Additional areas of the brain that process desires and rewards have been shown to differ between those with high and low self-control. Thus, those with high self-control have higher activity in the prefrontal cortex and lower activity in the desire and reward areas of the brain. It would seem that this type of brain activity may be present early in life, as illustrated by a now famous test called the marshmallow test.

In the marshmallow test, preschoolers sat in a room alone for a matter of minutes. One by one the preschoolers sat at a table with treats such as marshmallows on a plate. Before leaving the child alone, the researcher told each child that if they could wait until the researcher returned, they could have two marshmallows, but if they could not wait, then they could have only one marshmallow. Some ate the single marshmallow immediately, but approximately one third of the preschoolers were able to delay gratification long enough to get two marshmallows, which leaves two thirds unable to wait long enough even if they didn't eat the marshmallow immediately. Decades later, another group of researchers found nearly 60 of the original marshmallow-test preschoolers, who were now adults, and found that those who struggled to resist temptation as a preschooler showed similar scores on a test of self-control as an adult, and those who were able to resist temptation as a preschooler scored high on the self-control test as an adult.

In addition to the possibility that our self-control abilities or our willpower may be something we have more or less of from a very young age, other researchers have found that willpower is not an unlimited resource, leading them to coin the term willpower depletion. They say that willpower is like a muscle in your body. When you use your muscles to the point that the muscle group becomes fatigued, you cannot use those muscles effectively any more or at all. Similarly, when you have to repeatedly delay gratification or resist temptation, eventually your ability to do so will get fatigued. You may really want to resist, and you may exert a lot of effort trying to do so, but if you have already overused your ability to exert self-control, then you will find subsequent attempts are likely to fail and you will not be able to resist temptation, regardless of what your long-term goals are. Interestingly, however, researchers have concluded that regularly exerting self-control can help strengthen this ability. Just as when growing muscles repeated use over time results in larger or well-toned muscles, the key is to not overdo it in one day or one session and completely deplete one's self-control.

The reality is that we experience a multitude of things that can deplete our willpower, such as maintaining interpersonal relationships. A variety of studies have shown that people who, for example, were asked to suppress their feelings during a movie with strong emotional themes, or who were asked to convince a hostile audience that they were likeable, performed poorly on a later test of self-control. Sometimes, willpower can be restored after refueling the brain. Researchers have found that those who exert a lot of willpower have lower glucose (i.e., blood sugar) levels compared to those who exerted less willpower; however, when the subjects drank either sugared lemonade or sugar-free lemonade, those who drank lemonade with sugar restored some willpower. Additionally, other researchers have identified the importance of one's beliefs and attitudes when it comes to engaging in behavior. They found that those who exert self-control for their own reasons were able to sustain self-control much longer than those who engaged their willpower because others want them to (e.g., someone important to you tells you that you should lose weight, so you try to lose weight for them).

In terms of resisting foods that are associated with weight gain and increased fat deposits, the willpower-depletion model applies directly and has been studied by numerous researchers. Not surprisingly, researchers have found that children able to engage in self-control were less likely to become overweight as adolescents due to their ability to resist immediate temptation. However, as noted previously in this answer, the more someone exerts self-control, the less likely they will be able to resist the next temptation that comes along. The study that asked some movie watchers to suppress their emotional reactions when watching a highly emotional movie (whereas others were allowed to express whatever emotions they felt) found that these same moviegoers ate more ice cream immediately following the movie compared to those who were allowed to feel freely. Moreover, researchers have specifically studied the reasons why someone may resist dessert food and found that those who resisted for their own reasons, compared to those who may have resisted in order to please the experimenter, performed better on a subsequent test of self-control.

The Harvard University School of Public Health produced a document entitled *Obesity Prevention Source: Food and Diet* that identifies types and quantities of food that can make it easier for someone to resist foods that are usually associated with weight gain. Choosing the healthier types and quantities of foods still requires the use of willpower if these behaviors are not already in place and/or "easy" for the individual. Researchers examining the self-control literature to determine, in part, when differences in trait self-control (i.e., self-control is characteristic of that person) truly affect behavior, found that differences in trait self-control are not important when it comes to dieting (which requires a great deal of delaying gratification). Rather, they found that trait self-control matters most when people want to form or break specific habits, or perform well at school or work. This means that self-control itself may not be the reason why some people are able to lose weight and others are not. Some researchers have explicitly called for moving the focus away from individual willpower since it is not an unlimited resource and it may not be as important a factor as previously believed, and moving the focus to overall health. They suggest focusing on making changes to the environment that result in less willpower needed to engage in healthy behaviors. For example, in one study, researchers slowed the speed of an elevator by only six seconds, which resulted in elevator usage cut by half. Thus, participants engaged in more physical activity simply by not using the elevator by their own choice.

Finally, another study found that among those who were obese, only those who reported having limited self-control showed lower well-being compared to obese individuals who stated they had high self-control. This adds to the notion that it may not be actual self-control that matters when it comes to behaviors and well-being, but one's perception of their level of self-control. These researchers conceded that the easy availability of unhealthy foods and drinks negatively impacts those who believe they have little self-control, thus echoing other researcher's calls for environmental changes that require less effort to make healthy choices.

❖❖❖

Consequences

20. What diseases are linked to obesity?

There are myriad diseased linked to obesity. Before getting into specifics about the various diseases, it is important to note the distinction between one thing being linked to another and one thing causing something else. The vast majority of research in the area of disease and obesity are correlational research studies. These types of studies examine connections, or links, between two or more items of interest—in this case the two items are obesity and a specific disease. Finding a link between two things tells us only that if one thing exists the other thing is also more likely to exist (e.g., if someone is obese, they are more likely to have a specific disease). Correlational studies, however, do not provide information about whether or not obesity causes the disease or if there is something else that may be the cause of the disease or, alternatively, the cause of both obesity and the disease (see Questions 9–19 for information about factors related to obesity). The diseases that are often linked to obesity are diabetes, cardiovascular disease, cancer, sleep apnea, nonalcoholic fatty liver disease, and osteoarthritis.

There is more than one form of diabetes; however, the type that is most commonly linked to obesity is type 2 diabetes mellitus. The research examining this relationship has found that as someone's body mass index (BMI) increases (see Questions 1 and 2 for more information about BMI), their risk for developing type 2 diabetes also increases. Those who are classified as overweight according to BMI are two to five times more likely to develop type 2 diabetes compared to those with a lower BMI. For those who have a BMI of 35 or higher, the risk for developing type 2 diabetes skyrockets to 42–93 times greater than those with a lower BMI.

Diabetes is a disease that develops as a result of a problem with the body's inability to effectively use or make insulin, which is important for moderating the amount of blood sugar (i.e., glucose) someone has. Someone who has type 1 diabetes has a body that cannot manufacture insulin and, therefore, requires insulin injections. The body of someone with type 2 diabetes can make insulin but is unable to use it effectively and is, therefore, more likely to develop hyperglycemia, which occurs when there is too much glucose in the bloodstream. Some studies have shown that the risk of developing type 2 diabetes, which is greater in those who are overweight or obese, seems to be connected to the amount of upper body fat someone has, such that the more upper body fat the person has, the more likely they will be to develop type 2 diabetes (see also Question 5 for more information about metabolic syndrome).

Cardiovascular disease is a generic term referring to problems with the heart and blood vessels. Though it is possible to be born with a risk for developing problems with one's cardiovascular system, for most people the causes are more within our control. Things such as smoking, types of food consumed, and regularity of exercise are usually changeable. Being overweight or obese have also been identified as risk factors for cardiovascular disease. The link between one's body weight and cardiovascular disease has been described as being the result of an increase in blood volume due to having a larger body size. The more blood found in one's body, the more the heart has to work to pump the blood, which can lead to hypertension, or enlargement of the heart's left ventricle. These issues can then further compromise the heart's ability to function adequately, leading to more problems with the cardiovascular system. Obese adults who are less than 50 years old have a 2–2.5 times greater chance of developing coronary heart disease than those with a lower BMI. Overall, studies have found that as one's BMI increases, the risk for developing a problem with one's cardiovascular system also increases.

There are many different types of cancer, and not all are linked to body size. Those that typically are include (but are not limited to) endometrial cancer, liver cancer, kidney cancer, colorectal cancer, breast cancer, and thyroid cancer. Factors such as degree of inflammation in the body, how much fatty tissue the body has, and the body's insulin level have been linked to the development of cancer. Uncontrolled inflammation in the body can alter one's DNA and change the rate of cell growth, which puts someone at greater risk for developing cancer. Additionally, higher amounts of fatty tissue in the body have also been linked to cancer. Although some amount of fatty tissue, particularly for women, has health benefits, too much can result in too much estrogen being produced, which has been linked to certain types of cancer (e.g., breast cancer). Higher insulin levels can result in diabetes as well as some forms of cancer.

Getting adequate sleep on a regular basis is routinely identified as an important factor in maintaining and improving one's health. Thus, problems with one's ability to get enough quality sleep is not only a nuisance but can also be an indication of a serious problem. There are two types of sleep apnea: obstructive sleep apnea and central sleep apnea. Regardless of the type, sleep apnea is a disorder diagnosed when someone stops breathing while they are sleeping. In obstructive sleep apnea, the cessation of breathing occurs because soft tissue in the back of the throat collapses and interferes with one's airway, thereby preventing them from breathing properly or at all. In central sleep apnea, the brain itself is not functioning properly and does not tell the body to breathe as it should. Regardless of the type of sleep apnea, the individual dealing with it will eventually wake up and breathe again; however, the cycle of continuously stopping breathing and waking up to start breathing significantly impacts the quality and quantity of sleep one gets. Although sleep apnea can be diagnosed in individuals regardless of body size, it is likely that those with larger bodies and more body fat will be at greater risk for developing this sleep disorder.

Another disorder associated with body fat is nonalcoholic fatty liver disease (NAFLD). Fatty liver disease refers to an excess accumulation of fat in the liver and is usually associated with alcoholism. In the case of NAFLD, alcohol is not involved. As many as 15 percent of nonobese people can be diagnosed with NAFLD whereas upwards of 85 percent of those who are classified at the highest level of obesity may be diagnosed with NAFLD. The American Liver Foundation states that risk factors for developing NAFLD include diabetes, poor eating habits, and losing weight in a short amount of time. Symptoms of metabolic syndrome (see Question 5 for more information about this syndrome) have been connected to NAFLD as well as obesity; however, as many as 30 percent of those who are obese do not have metabolic syndrome. Thus, although there may be a link between NAFLD and obesity, the nature of the connection seems to be unclear.

Osteoarthritis is a joint disease that is a common issue for many people regardless of body size. This type of arthritis is often referred to as "wear and tear" arthritis and often results in stiffness in the joints after a period

of not using them (e.g., when sitting) and pain. Although not life threatening, osteoarthritis can negatively impact one's quality of life and
can result in becoming sedentary, which can then contribute to the development of things such as diabetes or heart disease. Although the nick-
name for this type of arthritis is wear and tear, arthritis research has
since found that wear and tear alone does not account for all cases.
Genetic traits and injury can also account for the development of this
form of arthritis. One's weight has also been linked to osteoarthritis, particularly in major joints such as hips and knees, such that the more one
weighs, the more pressure is placed on these joints, which can ultimately
contribute to the breakdown in cartilage leading to the development of
osteoarthritis.

21. What mental health issues are linked to obesity?

Mental health issues that have been linked to obesity tend not to have a
direct connection to body size in and of itself. That is, there are other factors that seem to better explain why those who are overweight or obese
may be more likely to develop certain mental health issues. The primary
mitigating factor is anti-fat bias, also known as weight stigma or weight
discrimination (see Question 7 for more information about anti-fat bias).

Research has found that those who routinely experience anti-fat bias
are more likely to have both physical and mental health problems. In fact,
those who experience anti-fat bias are more likely to have self-esteem
issues, suffer from depression and some forms of anxiety, have higher levels of body dissatisfaction, and, for some, have higher rates of behaviors
associated with an eating disorder (i.e., anorexia nervosa, bulimia nervosa, binge eating disorder). One study found that as many as 50 percent
of those who experience anti-fat bias and who are overweight or obese can
be diagnosed with a mental health disorder such as depression, anxiety, or
a substance-use disorder. This study found that it was the stress of experiencing weight-related discrimination rather than one's weight that
explained the presence of the mental health issue. These researchers also
found that even really good social support (e.g., love and care from friends
and family) did not protect these individuals from experiencing the negative impact of anti-fat bias.

Some researchers have stated that the effect anti-fat bias can have on
those who are overweight or obese is significant enough that it should be
considered a public health issue. These researchers echoed the findings of
others in that when they examined data such as someone's BMI, their age

when they became obese, their age at the time of the study, and their sex, they found that none of these variables explained the high prevalence of mental health issues such as low self-esteem (which in and of itself can lead to more serious mental health concerns) or clinical depression. The variable that did offer an explanation was the individuals' experience with anti-fat bias.

Another factor that may be implicated in the presence of mental health issues among those who experience anti-fat bias is the internalization of this type of bias. Internalization of anti-fat bias or weight stigma means that someone who is overweight or obese will adopt an anti-fat bias themselves and view larger bodies, including their own, negatively. Interestingly, this type of internalization seems to occur more frequently among those who are obese or overweight. Individuals from other marginalized groups based on things such as race or religion tend not to adopt the negative beliefs others have about members of their particular group. In fact, the opposite seems to occur. When individuals from other groups experience negative stigmatic beliefs, they are more likely to view other members of their group more favorably. Researchers concluded that an explanation for this difference may be found in the belief that one's weight is under one's control and should be changed if one's weight is too high. Thus, not weighing the "right" amount is viewed as a personal failure, and any failed attempts to lose weight confirm for the individual that he or she is a bad person who is also lazy, which further leads them to think that they deserve the negative views they and others have about them. The significant impact that internalization of weight stigma can have on one's overall psychological well-being has led some to suggest that this phenomenon should be a specific focus for any plan or program designed to improve someone's psychological health.

22. How does obesity affect one's relationships with family and friends?

This is a complex question that involves one's own perception about one's own body as well as the perception that friends and family have about one's body. Specifically, this boils down to the presence or lack of anti-fat bias (see Questions 7 and 8 for information about anti-fat bias and body acceptance). As a reminder, anti-fat bias, otherwise known as weight stigma or weight discrimination, refers to the negative beliefs about and attitudes toward someone who is overweight or obese. When these attitudes and beliefs are present in friends and family, there will likely be a negative impact not only on that individual's well-being (see Question 21 for information about mental health issues and obesity) but also on the relationships themselves. Those with family and friends who believe that individuals who are obese or overweight can easily change their body size if they just put in enough effort and exert enough willpower (see Question 19 for more information about willpower and obesity) are likely to routinely hear comments about their weight, advice about weight loss, and perhaps harsh criticism about what their body looks like and who they are as a person. Such beliefs can inevitably strain these relationships, particularly if the individual who is overweight or obese has worked really hard at trying to control their weight and to lose weight permanently but ultimately gained the weight back. Some individuals may hear comments from friends and family about what they're eating or hints about what may happen if they eat what they are about to eat (e.g., "Are you sure you want to eat that?" "That's only going to make you fatter."). Comments such as these are often intended to be well meaning but can ultimately leave the person feeling ashamed, embarrassed, and unsure of what to do at mealtimes.

By contrast, if anti-fat bias has been internalized (i.e., the person themselves views fat bodies, including their own, and fat people negatively), relationships with friends and family can still suffer even if their loved ones do not have anti-fat bias themselves. Those who internalize anti-fat bias may reject supportive comments and efforts by those who care about them. They may not believe they deserve positive attention and, in fact, may believe they deserve to be ridiculed or made to feel ashamed. This can leave loved ones feeling frustrated that their supportive efforts are rejected, which can result in the loved ones' pulling away physically and emotionally or trying even harder to convince the person that they are worthy of love and respect. Either way, the relationship is likely to be strained.

Regardless of in whom the anti-fat bias exists, the result of experiencing it can diminish one's overall well-being and may lead to psychological problems such as depression, anxiety, or eating disorders (see Question 21 for more information about mental health issues and obesity). This can further strain important relationships since the presence of mental illness is known to significantly impact family and friends as they do not always know what to do to be helpful and may become frustrated or even angry that the person dealing with a mental illness is not showing signs of getting better. Feelings of helplessness among loved ones, depending on their severity and intensity, can negatively impact the overall well-being of the loved one themselves, leaving them less able to be supportive.

When none involved hold an anti-fat bias, there is a much greater chance that the impact obesity has on these relationships is nonexistent. All involved will likely view one another in terms of who they are rather than what size their body is, which may lead to stronger and more positive relationships.

23. What are the costs to society at large due to obesity?

When obesity is discussed in terms of what it costs society at large to have a significant portion of the population classified as obese, the conversation inevitably settles on the rising cost of health insurance and healthcare in general. The argument is that the reason insurance rates and medical procedures cost more than they ever have (taking inflation into account) is, in part, due to the fact that obese people are more likely to experience serious medical conditions (see Question 20 for information about diseases linked to obesity) and, therefore, require more medical care than their normal-weight counterparts. The greater use of medical services means that insurance companies are likely having to pay more for these services and, therefore, pass along these costs to all who purchase health insurance. This is decried as unfair by those who are not obese.

Some researchers have examined this issue and have come to the conclusion that due to the serious medical issues associated with obesity, there is an overall decrease in lifespan (see Question 25 for more information about lifespan and obesity), a decline in work-related productivity, and a decision to retire earlier. Each of these in and of themselves has the potential to negatively impact society at large; if healthcare costs are passed along to others, others have to work harder to pick up the slack for those who aren't being productive or who leave work for retirement earlier than expected. Other researchers, however, have refuted these conclusions, citing findings that show that those in the upper end of the normal weight and all of the overweight categories may live longer than those in all other BMI categories, that those using healthcare services the least are found in the overweight category, that a significant proportion of those in the normal-weight category were found to be metabolically unhealthy, which can lead to many of the serious medical issues associated with obesity (see Question 5 for more information about metabolic syndrome), and that an even higher percentage of those who were classified as overweight or obese were found to be metabolically healthy. Thus, the conclusions these researchers made was that BMI is likely not a good indicator of one's risk with respect to health and healthcare costs.

Another type of insurance that has been found to be impacted by body size is worker's compensation. Some research has found that the higher someone's BMI, the more likely it is that they will miss work and that the employer may incur more costs overall. Findings such as these have resulted in some companies implementing policies targeting those with higher BMIs or offering incentives to those with lower BMIs. Other research has questioned the findings of previous work-related research, stating that one factor not examined was the degree to which the individual's job was sedentary. Recent research in this area has found that being sedentary overall can have a devastating impact on one's overall health and well-being and may, therefore, result in more days off work and/or the need for increased medical care. The implication is that it may not be body size but the degree to which someone is active that may explain missed workdays and costs related to worker's compensation.

Another area related to body size that has been identified as having a burden on at least part of society is airline travel. It is known to many that airlines regulate how heavy one's baggage can be, and if your bag weighs more than their maximum standard, then the air traveler has to pay more to have their bag flown to their destination. The idea is that more weight results in greater fuel costs, and that cost is ultimately passed along to the consumer. This argument is, in part, what is used in the context of the increased cost of air travel. Some have argued that heavier people should pay more because they weigh more, resulting in higher fuel costs; others contend that if a larger-bodied person takes up space in a fellow passenger's seat, then the fellow passenger's rights have been infringed upon. These issues have led some to call for specific guidelines and policies when it comes to overweight or obese passengers. Some airlines do require obese passengers who cannot fit comfortably in a single seat to pay for a second seat. By contrast, advocates for larger-bodied travelers have stated that airlines should do more to ensure all passengers, regardless of body size (including height), are comfortable using the accommodations they have paid for.

24. Do insurance companies change healthcare coverage depending on whether or not someone is obese?

Although health insurance companies provide assistance with the cost of medical care, the reason they do so is because someone has purchased their insurance at a particular rate that guarantees them a particular type of healthcare coverage. Thus, insurance companies are businesses interested in profits and losses just as other businesses are. Insurance companies, like any other business, will look for ways to minimize costs while maximizing profits. One way they do this is to identify those who may be at greater risk for injury or disease which is therefore likely to result in more costly medical care. For example, smoking is typically identified as a high-risk behavior in terms of one's overall health, and insurance companies may, therefore, elect to charge smokers more for the same coverage that a non-smoker might have. This can also be the case for those who engage in other risky behaviors such as skydiving or rock climbing. The common denominator for these examples is that the behaviors are choices that the individual has elected. Insurance companies reason that if one chooses to put their life at risk, they should pay more for insurance coverage since it is more likely that they will need to use their insurance benefits (i.e., the insurance pays for some or all of a medical procedure) compared to those who do not engage in those behaviors. Obesity has become a similar concern in that several serious medical diseases are linked to obesity (see Question 20 for more information about diseases linked to obesity); additionally, the prevailing belief of many people—including healthcare providers and those who are obese themselves—that body size is a choice (see Question 19 for information about willpower and obesity) leads to the conclusion that the healthcare of obese people should be reduced or that the health insurance of obese people should cost more, as it does for smokers or skydivers.

As noted in Question 23, some researchers have specifically advocated for insurance companies to include BMI into their calculations for the cost of health insurance given the association between obesity and multiple medical issues Many insurance companies do, in fact, use BMI (see Questions 1 and 2 for more information about BMI and its classifications) to calculate their insurance premium rates (i.e., how much you pay for your health insurance). An article published by AIG, a life-insurance company, entitled *How Does BMI Affect Life Insurance Rates* noted that exceptions to the use of BMI may be made for those such as athletes who have a higher muscle-to-fat ratio and, therefore, may have a misleading BMI since muscle weighs more than fat by volume; however, the article did not note an exception for those who may have a high BMI in the absence of a high muscle ratio but who can also show that other indicators of their overall health are well within the range similar to those who do not have a high BMI. As other researchers have found, BMI may not be an adequate variable to consider for health risk. Nonetheless, BMI is used to calculate health (and death) risk. Those who fall into higher BMI categories such as overweight or obese may pay more for the same insurance coverage compared to someone else who is effectively identical in every other way except weight.

25. Do obese people live shorter lives?

The notion that those who are obese will live shorter lives is bolstered by the consistent findings linking obesity to a variety of serious medical problems (see Question 20 for more information about diseases linked to obesity). The idea is that if those who are obese are more likely to develop serious medical issues that can result in one's death, then they must be more likely to die sooner than those who are not obese and, therefore, at less risk for developing these same medical issues. Complicating the issue is the notion of whether or not life expectancy may be affected to a greater degree by the presence (or absence) of metabolic syndrome (see Question 5 for more information about metabolic syndrome), which can be present in anyone at any body size.

One article published in the late 2000s examined nearly 60 previously conducted studies on the connection between mortality and body size. Collectively, these studies had data on nearly 900,000 adults. The conclusion the authors drew was that the lowest mortality rate was found among adults classified in the middle of the normal-weight range (i.e., BMI between 22.5 and 25; see Question 2 for more information about BMI classifications). They also found, however, that for every five BMI points above this range there was a 30 percent greater chance of death for any reason. A similar conclusion was drawn for those who were classified in the underweight category according to BMI. That is, the lower one's BMI in the underweight category, the higher the risk for death. These authors acknowledged that BMI was not an ideal measure of how and where body fat is stored. They suggested that the mortality rate is likely higher among those in the overweight and obese categories. A study conducted several years after this one, however, seems to call into question this final conclusion.

In 2016, a study was published that looked at all-cause mortality rates (i.e., death due to any cause) over a period of nearly 40 years from 1976 to 2013. This study's results showed that the BMI of the group that had the lowest mortality rate has increased over the years. During the 1970s those with a BMI of 23.7 (normal range) had the lowest all-cause mortality rate. In the 1990s the group with the lowest all-cause mortality rate had risen to a BMI of 24.6 (normal rage), but in the 2000s and 2010s the group with the lowest all-cause mortality rate had a BMI of 27.0, which is considered to be pre-obese. Although the explanation for this rise is not clear, the authors speculated that improvements in healthcare and targeted public health campaigns on issues such as smoking and increasing physical activity may explain this trend. Additional research has found that those with a BMI of 35 or higher (a BMI of 30 classifies someone as obese; see Questions 1 and 2 for more information about BMI and its classifications) are at greater risk for all-cause mortality than those in the normal range; however, the lowest range of obesity (BMI of 30–34) did not have a higher all-cause mortality rate than those in the normal range. Moreover, this study confirmed previous findings that those in the overweight BMI range had the lowest all-cause mortality rate.

An examination of the role metabolic health (see Question 5 for information about metabolic syndrome) may play in mortality rates showed that among those classified as obese, nearly one quarter were metabolically healthy, and one third of those in the normal BMI range were found to be metabolically unhealthy. Upon further examination of their data, these researchers found that those who were obese and metabolically healthy were at no greater risk for cardiovascular disease than their metabolically healthy nonobese counterparts. When, however, either those who were obese or not obese had two or more symptoms associated with metabolic syndrome, both groups were at greater risk for developing cardiovascular disease. These researchers stated that those who were obese and metabolically healthy were not only at less risk for cardiovascular disease but also at less risk for all-cause mortality compared to those who were metabolically unhealthy. This led them to conclude that it is not body fat, per se, that places one at greater risk for disease or death but the degree to which an individual is metabolically healthy.

Treatment Options

26. What lifestyle changes can someone make who is obese?

The most obvious lifestyle changes someone can make who is obese or who otherwise wants to lose weight relate to diet and exercise. In fact, many people who intend on losing weight often go on a diet of some kind that is usually restrictive in nature (see Question 12 for more information about dieting). They may also, or instead, engage in some form of physical activity for the purpose of burning calories and thereby losing weight. Those who already exercise are likely to increase the amount and intensity of their exercise in order to burn more calories. An increase in exercise and a restriction in how much and what kinds of foods someone eats usually result in weight loss; however, it is not always that straightforward. Most people (over 90 percent and up to 95 percent) cannot sustain a diet plan that is restrictive in nature. As a result, they will go off their diet and either resume what they were eating before the diet or in some cases may start eating more than what they were eating prior to dieting. This often results in weight gain that may leave the person weighing more than they did to begin with (see Questions 4 and 12 for information about yo-yo dieting). An additional factor that affects how one's body uses the food that one eats is genetics (see Question 10 for more information about genetics and obesity).

Not everyone has an efficient metabolism, which means that they will burn fewer calories than someone with a more efficient metabolism.

Additionally, how much and how consistently someone exercises and how much one eats can interact with one's genetics to affect one's metabolism, resulting in either "easy" weight loss or weight loss that is very difficult to achieve despite "doing everything right." Genetics, of course, cannot be manipulated very easily, and, therefore, trying to fight one's genetics is typically futile. Another factor that can affect one's weight is much more firmly under our control, and that is stress.

High amounts of stress are known to affect many things related to our health including sleep, cardiovascular functioning, gastrointestinal functioning, and other underlying processes that can make us appear unwell. Too much stress is often implicated in poor eating habits and the improper digesting of food, both of which can result in weight gain. Thus, managing one's stress is important not only for preventing things such as heart attack, stroke, or cancer but also for trying to change one's weight. It is, therefore, important for individuals to identify effective techniques to manage their overall stress. For some people, this may mean rearranging their life so that they have fewer stressors overall (e.g., getting rid of responsibilities that they don't need to have). Many people feel obligated to take on more than is realistic for them in order to please others, to look good to their boss, and so on. For others, it may not be a matter of eliminating stressors so much as learning how to effectively cope with stress. As the saying goes, it is not the event or situation but our reaction to it that causes problems. Learning how to keep things in perspective and not make things more difficult than they need to be can be important skills to develop. This can be done by asking others how they manage stress or by seeking formal assistance through counseling or psychotherapy (see Questions 27 and 28 for more information about counseling and psychotherapy and their effectiveness with treating obesity).

Stress is inevitable. Regardless of whether someone is able to take on fewer responsibilities or perceive their obligations differently, stress of some form or another will persist, and it is, therefore, important to make time for activities that are purely enjoyable and serve no other purpose. This means that carving out leisure time or time you can devote to whatever you want means you'll have time to read a book, watch a movie, enjoy your pets, play with your children, take a long bath or shower, and so on. These activities when done for enjoyment or relaxation can be highly beneficial for one's overall health. And in the current context, the reduction of stress regardless of how it is managed can mean that one's weight-loss efforts are more manageable even if one does not lose the amount of weight one was hoping to (see Question 8 for information about body acceptance and the Health at Every Size® approach).

27. What types of counseling or psychotherapy are used to treat obesity?

The forms of counseling and psychotherapy that are often identified as being effective for the treatment of obesity are those that focus on helping people change their behaviors. Usually this means that the focus is helping people change what and how much they eat as well as how much they engage in physical activity. Other forms of counseling or psychotherapy will address the emotional state of the individual. Emotions commonly identified as "negative" (e.g., anger, sadness) are often associated with poor eating habits and can also be associated with stress (see Question 26 for more information about lifestyle changes), which can further be associated with weight loss or weight gain. Regardless of the type of counseling or psychotherapy in which someone may take part, this type of treatment is usually recommended before other, more invasive forms of treatment are tried (see Questions 29–32 for information about weight-loss medications and weight-loss surgery).

Behavior management refers to treatment that focuses on what a person does (i.e., what behaviors they engage in) as well as the degree to which their behaviors are helpful or harmful. Behavior-management strategies associated with obesity are typically focused on weight loss and ultimately weight-loss maintenance. Some forms of behavior-management counseling take place in the context of a diet program such as Jenny Craig® or Weight Watchers®. These programs outline parameters for participants to follow that usually involve rules and expectations around what food, how much food, and when foods can be eaten, as well as expectations or recommendations for physical activity. Counseling in the form of virtual or face-to-face support groups or individual meetings are also often part of these programs. The intent is to help participants stick to their plan, help them problem-solve dietary slips (e.g., eating something not on the diet plan), and get back on track.

Behavior management on an individual basis (as opposed to part of a commercial plan) is likely to take place between a counselor who may or may not be licensed to address mental health concerns. Since obesity and treating it through behavior management is not necessarily a mental health endeavor, it is legal and ethical for a non–mental health counselor to assist in this way. If, however, it is determined that a mental health issue is affecting one's ability to address food and physical activity concerns and/or an eating disorder is suspected, then a licensed mental health professional should become involved. Regardless of the professional's credentials, helping someone with behavior-management skills to address eating habits and physical activity will focus on identifying what the current behaviors are, what behaviors are desired, what the desired outcome is, what is getting in the way of someone's achieving that outcome, and what may ultimately support or reinforce the desired behaviors so they persist into the future. Success would, therefore, be defined as finding behaviors that result in weight loss that the individual can sustain over the long term.

In addition to pure behavior management, some forms of counseling may also include a focus on what the person is thinking and how they are feeling. Depending on the professional providing this type of counseling and what their particular approach is, the method used may be cognitive-behavioral therapy (CBT) or an in-depth, insight-oriented therapy such as psychodynamic psychotherapy. CBT primarily focuses the individual's thoughts and feelings to the extent that they affect desired and undesired behaviors—in this case, behaviors that facilitate weight loss and behaviors that interfere with this process. Psychodynamic psychotherapy is likely to focus more on the emotional experiences of the individual and to identify long-standing psychological patterns that may affect the individual negatively. The direct focus is not likely to be on weight loss per se but on what will help the individual improve their overall well-being and life satisfaction. In the context of treating obesity, success will still likely be defined as weight loss; however, throughout the process of in-depth, insight-oriented psychotherapy, the individual may shift their focus so that the goal is no longer weight loss but doing things that support their emotional, physical, and spiritual well-being, which will likely include engaging in health-enhancing behaviors such as eating well and engaging in regular physical activity.

Some professionals and community groups may take a Health at Every Size® approach (see Question 8 for more information about body acceptance and the Health at Every Size® approach), which will not focus on weight loss at all but will support the individual in doing things that are good for their overall health and well-being, as well as helping them to come to terms with the fact that their body size may not change as much as they would like (or at all) but that the healthy behaviors they are using will contribute to feeling and being healthier.

28. How effective is counseling or psychotherapy in treating obesity?

Since obesity is about BMI (see Questions 1 and 2 for more information about BMI and its classifications), which is reflected in the ratio between one's height and one's weight, the treatment of obesity is about lowering one's BMI, which would occur via weight loss. Thus, the question about how effective counseling or psychotherapy is in treating obesity is truly about how effective these treatment methods are for weight loss, presumably sustained weight loss. Anecdotally, most readers probably know many people who have lost weight (regardless of body size) either on their own, by following a particular program, and/or with the help of a counselor or psychotherapist. This usually leads people to conclude that weight loss is in fact possible and is a matter of willpower (see Question 19 for a discussion of willpower) and effort. A great deal of research supports the idea that weight loss is possible; however, there is a growing body of research suggesting that weight loss is possible in the short term but not likely in the long term. Additionally, some research has shown that when weight loss is sustained, it does not necessarily result in the change of someone's BMI classification.

Due to this nation's focus on obesity and the "obesity epidemic," professionals from myriad disciplines (e.g., psychology, medicine, nutrition) have devoted considerable resources to figuring out the most effective way to help people lose weight, prevent weight gain, and maintain a "healthy" weight. One result of this focus on weight is that there is a large body of literature examining what works and what doesn't when it comes to weight loss. Usually, when people do lose weight, their intent is to keep it off. Thus, researchers needed to define what constitutes meaningful weight loss and what period of time constitutes maintenance of that weight loss. Definitions have varied widely over the years, which prompted a group of researchers in the early 2000s to define meaningful weight loss as the loss of at least 10 percent of one's body weight, and maintenance of that weight loss would be considered achieved if it was sustained for at least one year—the one-year mark is often used as the definition for long-term weight loss in others' research. These same researchers developed the National Weight Control Registry (NWCR) in the mid-1990s. This registry has over 10,000 participants who are admitted if they have lost at least 30 pounds and kept that weight off for at least one year. Overall, the collective results of these individuals' experiences is that they have lost, on average, 66 pounds and kept that weight off for over five years. One commonality among nearly 90 percent of those in the registry is that they had tried and failed at previous weight-loss attempts, and what seemed to make them successful this time was that they were more likely to emphasize physical activity in their efforts. Additionally, they were likely to change how they ate, such that they consumed fewer calories, eliminated some types of food from their diets, and generally kept track of how much they ate. Although the experiences of those in the NWCR are promising and seem to point to long-term weight loss, critics of such a conclusion indicate that although 10,000 people is a lot, it is a small fraction of those who have tried to lose weight and who may not have had the success that those in the registry have had. Thus, these critics say that those in the registry are not likely representative of the typical individual trying to lose weight.

Additional studies have also examined sustained weight loss in an attempt to determine what constitutes successful weight loss. One set of authors examined a variety of previously published studies that had been conducted on weight loss to determine if one method of weight loss was more successful than another. They concluded that changing how one eats in combination with engaging in physical activity resulted in more weight loss than doing one or the other. When both diet and exercise were addressed, individuals were likely to keep the weight off for one year. These same researchers, however, noted that among all participants, 50 percent of whatever weight they lost had been regained regardless of how they achieved their weight loss. Another article examining multiple studies on weight loss looked at the overall effectiveness of making behavioral changes, taking weight-loss medication (see Questions 29 and 30 for more about weight-loss medications), or having weight-loss surgery (see Questions 31 and 32 for more information about weight-loss surgery/bariatric surgery). They found that weight loss ranged from 11 pounds (behavioral changes) to upwards of 165 pounds (weight-loss surgery), with weight loss associated with medication ranging between 11 and 22 pounds. Additionally, this weight was kept off for one to four years depending in part on the weight-loss method, but also how long the researchers tracked the study participants. Other studies echoed these findings in that weight loss did occur among many, but not all, study participants and that it was sustained for at least one year, leading them to conclude that weight loss is possible and worth attempting.

Other researchers, however, have challenged these conclusions, stating that the definition of long-term weight loss as weight that has been kept off for at least one year is not truly long-term weight loss. Certainly, some studies demonstrated that some participants sustained weight loss for more than one year and as long as four years; however, critics of the notion that long-term weight loss is possible based on a one-year timeline have suggested that sustained weight loss over a period of at least five years is a more reasonable definition of long-term weight loss. In addition to challenging what constitutes long-term weight loss, some of these researchers also question the pursuit of weight loss to begin with. Some studies revealed that weight-loss efforts can actually result in weight gain. In an attempt to understand why this might occur, one study examined the dieting behavior of adolescents and found that weight gain was the most likely result, which they found was probably due to the nature of going on a diet to begin with. Going on a diet implies that one will go off that diet at some point; thus, the dieting behaviors are likely to be extreme (e.g., severe restriction in calories). One byproduct of this seemed to be binge-eating behavior following the dieting behavior, which is then associated with an increase in weight (and BMI) over time.

Another group of researchers examined the soundness of previous weight-loss research, particularly those studies that concluded that long-term weight loss is possible and that it leads to health benefits. After examining numerous studies and applying a rigorous standard to those studies and their interpretations, this research group concluded that although weight loss was demonstrated in these studies, the longer the participants were followed, the more weight was gained. They also stated that studies concluding that weight loss is possible and leads to improved health reported that weight loss did not typically result in a change in BMI category. Moreover, it was unclear whether it was weight loss per se that contributed to improved health markers rather than things like positive changes in physical activity, less alcohol consumption, lower sodium consumption, and so on. Overall, this research group concluded that the benefits associated with weight loss are small and that it is unclear that the benefits are the result of weight loss directly. They also concluded that yo-yo dieting (see Questions 4 and 12 for more information) and its associated medical problems can occur since many of those studied who lost weight gained it back plus additional pounds. Their final conclusion was that the benefits of weight loss do not outweigh the possible risks, and thus weight loss should not be recommended as a form of treatment for obesity.

29. What types of medications are used to treat obesity?

Medications used to treat obesity are also referred to as weight-loss medications. As is the case with bariatric surgery (see Questions 31 and 32 for more information about this form of treatment), the prescription of weight-loss medications is based on the patient's BMI (see Questions 1 and 2 for more information about BMI). Some medications have the requirement that patients have a BMI of at least 27 and others a BMI of at least 30. There are no weight-loss medications approved for use in the United States for children younger than 12 years old. Regardless of age or

BMI, when these medications are prescribed, they are usually done so in conjunction with rather than in place of behavioral methods of treatment (see Questions 27 and 28 for more information about treatment via counseling or psychotherapy). Additionally, like any other prescription medication, weight-loss medications may not work for everyone, and for some, the side effects of the medication may supersede any weight loss that results.

Weight-loss medications are designed to do one of two things: alter the cues we receive for hunger and fullness, or inhibit the body's absorption of fat. Several medications have been approved by the U.S. Food and Drug Administration (FDA) for the purpose of weight loss. None of the approved medications are approved for lifetime use, although some are approved for use over the course of many months or years. Only one medication is approved for nonadult patients, but they must be at least 12 years of age.

The medication known as orlistat, which has the trade names of Xenical® or Alli® (Alli® is an over-the-counter medication and thus does not require a prescription), is the only medication approved for use for individuals 12 years or older. All other medications are approved only for adults. Orlistat works in the body by preventing fat from being absorbed, meaning that most fat consumed via food will not be fully digested and will ultimately be expelled by the body. This explains some of the medication's side effects, which include stomach pain, gas, diarrhea, and leakage of oily stools.

The medication lorcaserin (trade name Belviq®) operates by affecting the chemicals found in the brain called neurotransmitters. Specifically, lorcaserin affects the neurotransmitter serotonin, which is known to affect one's mood, sleep, memory, sexual interest, and appetite and digestion. Patients for whom lorcaserin is effective will feel full after eating small amounts of food and thus will consume less food overall. Lorcaserin can interact with other medications and, therefore, must be used with caution, especially if the patient is taking another medication that affects serotonin. Side effects of this medication include headaches, dizziness, fatigue, nausea, or constipation.

Penermine-topiramate (trade name Qsymia®) combines two different drugs. One of the drugs causes a decrease in people's appetite and desire to eat. The other drug induces feelings of fullness and also causes food to not be as appealing. The overall effect, of course, is that the individual will eat less food while taking this medication. Side effects for penermine-topiramate include tingling sensations, dizziness, difficulty sleeping, constipation, and a change in taste. This particular medication is not recommended for women who are pregnant or who are trying to become pregnant as it can cause birth defects.

The remaining four medications—phentermine, bezphetamine, diethylpropion, and phendimetrazine—are controlled substances due to their potential for addiction. Therefore, these medications are prescribed only for short-term use. Collectively, these medications affect one's appetite so that one either feels not hungry or feels full. Some other medications may be prescribed for off-label use but are not approved by the FDA for weight loss. What this means is that these medications are approved for and often prescribed for some other issues (e.g., depression) and may have the side effect of weight loss. Thus, a medication like this may be prescribed, off-label, for weight loss.

As with any treatment that may affect how one's body functions, it is always important to fully consult with one's primary care provider (or specialist) about taking any of these medications and to learn as much about them as possible.

30. How effective are weight-loss medications?

As noted in Question 29, weight-loss medications do not work for everyone. Sometimes it is a matter of finding the right medication at the right dose; however, for some patients, there may not be any FDA-approved medications that result in meaningful weight loss. In this regard, for some patients, weight-loss medications are not effective. Other patients may see meaningful weight loss as a result of a prescribed weight-loss medication; therefore, it is correct to say that for these patients, weight-loss medications are effective. Those for whom weight-loss medications are effective can expect to lose around 10 percent of their body weight, which is likely to occur during the first six months of taking the medication. After that, weight loss would be predicted to slow down, and some individuals may experience weight gain. Another consideration with regard to effectiveness has to do with how long someone can take any of these medications. Prescribed weight-loss medications may be approved for use over the course of years; however, for many people, the prescription is intended to be for shorter-term use such as several months. Additionally, some weight-loss medications are potentially addictive and are, therefore, approved only for shorter-term use. This means, of course, that no weight-loss medications are intended to be used for nor are they FDA approved for lifetime use. This begs the question: What happens when the medication is discontinued? The answer is that weight-loss medications are not intended to be the only form of treatment.

When prescribed a weight-loss medication, it is typically the case that the patient is also taking part in some form of behavioral health treatment involving counseling or psychotherapy (see Questions 27 and 28 for more information) likely focused on helping the patient change their eating habits, address stress and emotional concerns that may affect how much and what types of food they are eating, and change their level of exercise and physical activity. The implication is that when the medication is discontinued as planned, the patient will have developed sufficient skills so that they can continue to eat in a healthier way (compared to how they were eating before treatment), thereby either continuing to lose weight or maintaining what weight they have lost. Since some of these medications function by suppressing hunger cues and enhancing fullness cues, it is possible that while taking a weight-loss medication a patient may consume much less than what their body needs to function in a healthy way. One result of inadequate intake of calories is that the metabolism may slow. Thus, when the medication is discontinued, even when gradually taken off, hunger cues and fullness cues will likely return to normal. Even eating a normal, healthy amount of food may result in weight gain if a patient's metabolism has slowed enough that it is no longer burning calories as efficiently as prior to starting the medication regimen.

31. What are the different types of weight-loss or bariatric surgery?

Bariatric surgery is the formal name for weight-loss surgery. There are several different types of weight-loss surgery, some of which have been performed since the 1960s. Weight-loss surgery is performed only on adults who have a BMI of 35 or higher or 40 or higher depending on the procedure (see Questions 1 and 2 for more information about BMI). These types of surgeries are not typically recommended for children; however, some surgeries can be performed on children, though with more strict requirements than for adults.

Weight-loss surgery can be recommended by one's physician. Alternatively, the patient themselves may request a referral from their physician for the surgery. Regardless of who initiates the discussion, before any weight-loss surgery will be performed for any patient, they will typically go through an assessment and screening process to ensure that the patient is a viable candidate for surgery both physically and psychologically. A patient must be well enough in both regards for surgery to be effective and safe. As with any surgery, the patient needs to be free of physical illness or other risk factors that might make undergoing major surgery dangerous. Psychologically, patients must also be well enough. Patients are often assessed for the presence of an eating disorder or other mental illnesses that might make following through on post-surgery requirements more difficult. The presence of any mental illness that might compromise a patient in this way may be referred for counseling or psychotherapy to address these psychological concerns prior to surgery. Additionally, some surgeons may not agree to perform a weight-loss surgery until the patient can demonstrate they are capable of losing some weight on their own.

There are currently four types of weight-loss or bariatric surgery that in one way or another alter one's digestive system, thereby decreasing food intake or preventing food from being fully digested, the result of which is weight loss. The four types of surgery are the adjustable gastric band (AGB), Roux-en-Y gastric bypass (RYGB), biliopancreatic diversion with a duodenal switch (BPD-DS), and vertical sleeve gastrectomy (VSG). Each surgery can be performed laparoscopically or using an open approach. Surgery performed laparoscopically will require less healing time, and the chances of complications following surgery are much lower than surgeries performed using the open approach. Laparoscopic surgeries involve inserting surgical instruments into the body, via small incisions, to perform the procedure, whereas the open approach involves an incision large enough to reveal the entire digestive system. Laparoscopic surgery is usually the preferred method; however, not all patients are candidates for this approach, and some, therefore, require the open approach, resulting in a longer recovery time and being at greater risk for postsurgical complications.

The AGB procedure involves the surgeon's placing a band around the top portion of the stomach, making the opening between the bottom of the throat and the top of the stomach smaller than it naturally is, resulting in a decrease in food intake. The opening is made smaller via a balloon inside the band that is inflated or deflated as needed, resulting in the constriction or dilation of the opening, respectively. The size of the opening (based on how inflated the balloon is) is determined by the patient's weight-loss and nutritional needs—the smaller the opening, the less food can be taken into the body, resulting in more weight loss.

The RYGB procedure also restricts food intake but in a much different way. With this procedure, a small pouch is created at the top of the stomach—the remainder of the stomach is cut off from the digestive process as the pouch itself serves as the entire stomach. Thus, the remainder of the stomach and two other portions of the digestive system (duodenum and the upper intestine) are bypassed so food that makes it into the small pouch is rerouted directly to the small intestine. Weight

loss, therefore, occurs because only small amounts of food can be consumed at a time (since the stomach pouch is so small) and some parts of
the digestive system that begin the digestive process are bypassed and,
therefore, not processing food.

When a patient is a candidate for the BPD-DS procedure, their surgery
will involve removing a significant proportion of the stomach, leaving a
much smaller stomach. This results in the patient's feeling full much
sooner than they normally would, so they will eat less food at a time. This
procedure also diverts food around a portion of the small intestine, which
means that less food will be absorbed by the patient's body. The removal
of a large part of the stomach and the diversion of food around part of the
small intestine also means that the normal digestive process is affected
such that less food is fully digested, resulting in fewer calories absorbed by
the body.

The fourth procedure, the VSG, serves a similar purpose to the BPD-
DS in that food intake is restricted and the food that is eaten is not fully
digested or absorbed, resulting in weight loss. This is achieved by the surgeon's removing part of the stomach, leaving behind a tube-shaped section of the stomach (i.e., a sleeve) that is about the same diameter as the
small intestine.

Given the nature of weight-loss surgeries, that they are considered
major surgeries most of which result in the removal of some portion of
one's digestive system, it is recommended that prospective patients not
only fully understand the nature of the procedures themselves but also the
risks, consequences, and known side effects. Those who are candidates for
bariatric surgery and who elect to have one of the procedures done must
dramatically alter how they eat for the rest of their lives. This includes not
only how much food they can eat but also what foods they can eat. Some
foods can no longer be digested or cannot be digested properly, which can
cause discomfort at best and illness at worst. Additionally, patients who
have one of these procedures done usually have to take numerous supplements to ensure they get the proper vitamins and nutrients that they can
no longer absorb through consuming food.

32. How effective is bariatric surgery?

The short answer to this question is that bariatric surgery is effective
if considering whether or not people lose weight when they've had one
of these procedures performed on them. The longer and more complete answer is, of course, more complicated when taking into account

long-term weight loss, side effects, and the possibility that someone could die from surgery.

Side effects of these forms of surgery seem to range from somewhat irritating to potentially very serious. Common side effects that are also associated with other surgeries include internal bleeding, infection, and blood clots. These side effects are not necessarily a result of these specific procedures but are possible with major surgery of any kind. Some side effects, however, are directly linked to bariatric surgeries themselves. For example, patients who have a form of bariatric surgery that involves redesigning the digestive system can experience intestinal leakage at locations where the digestive tract is newly surgically sewn together. This can result in the development of an infection (including the infection of other organs), resulting in things such as pain in the abdomen, fever, diarrhea, infection of the bloodstream, and death. Assuming these surgical complications do not arise, it is possible for serious postsurgical complications to surface, including nervous system damage due to lack of proper nutrition that goes undiagnosed and untreated. Other side effects can include the development of a hernia, and something called a stricture, which, in this context, means that the location where the intestines are joined becomes narrower than it should be.

The most serious potential side effect of or consequence of bariatric surgery is death. Death is, of course, a risk for any major surgery; however, some studies have indicated that death closely following bariatric surgery is about 1–2 percent but increases as time passes and increases with the age of the patient to as high as 4.5–6 percent. Not all of these deaths are directly and immediately related to the surgery itself, and something such as coronary heart disease has been identified as one cause of death accounting for these numbers. It is unknown, however, if death for something like heart disease would have occurred regardless of this type of surgery or if it was brought about due to the nature of these surgeries and the way in which they alter how essential minerals and nutrients are (or are not) absorbed into the body.

Another wrinkle in the answer to the question of whether or not bariatric surgery is effective is in terms of how much weight is lost and whether or not that weight is kept off. Bariatric surgery is typically marketed to morbidly obese individuals and is identified as an effective treatment for this classification of obesity. The reality is, however, that although patients who elect to have bariatric surgery will lose weight, it is highly unlikely that the individual will lose enough weight to be no longer considered obese. It is, therefore, not a cure for obesity itself. Morbid obesity is routinely identified as being the unhealthiest category of obesity, so losing enough weight to no longer be categorized in this class of obesity may be beneficial, but bariatric surgery may not result in becoming normal weight or even overweight.

Finally, although bariatric surgery is designed to result in weight loss, these are not procedures that will prevent future weight gain. Some patients, of course, will lose weight and keep it off, whereas others will lose weight and gain some or all of it back. In some cases, patients may gain back more than they initially lost. Weight gain can be the result of some other underlying medical issue, but it can also be the result of eating more than recommended, which can eventually stretch out the smaller stomach section that was surgically created.

As with any elective surgical procedure, it is important to learn as much as one can about the procedures themselves, their risks, the side effects, and the potential for long-term consequences including death. It is also important to talk with one's medical and mental health providers to ensure that bariatric surgery is a good choice given one's health status, lifestyle, and long-term goals.

33. Should someone who is obese pursue treatment of their obesity if they are not experiencing any adverse health effects?

This is a good question that requires an answer that is unique to each person who asks it of themselves. Some forms of treatment have significant and potentially serious side effects (see Questions 28–32 for information related to weight-loss medications and weight-loss surgery), and others have fewer side effects and are potentially much less dangerous (see Questions 26–28 for information related to lifestyle changes, and counseling or psychotherapy).

There are many people, laypeople as well as healthcare providers, who will unequivocally state that if someone is obese, even if they are not experiencing any adverse health effects that have been linked to obesity, they should receive some form of weight-loss treatment immediately. The thinking is that it will only be a matter of time before those adverse health effects appear. Some research does indicate that the higher one's obesity classification (see Questions 1 and 2 for more information about BMI and BMI classifications), the more likely they are to be diagnosed with serious health issues such as diabetes, heart disease, some forms of cancer, and so on. There are no studies, however, showing that all obese people of any classification will develop these adverse health effects. Moreover, the nature of the research shows that these medical issues are, in fact, linked to obesity but not necessarily caused by obesity (see Question 5 for information about metabolic syndrome). Of course, the seriousness of these medical conditions prompts many to take the stance that someone who is obese should not gamble that they will be among those who do not develop any of these problems. Research has found that those who take care of their bodies via regular physical activity and a healthy diet tend to be physically and psychologically healthy regardless of BMI classification in comparison to those who do not routinely exercise or eat in a healthy way (regardless of BMI classification). This may be good news to some but may also confuse those trying to decide what they should do. As with the other research, however, these findings are not true for 100 percent of people.

Realistically, there is no hard and fast rule as to who should seek weight-loss treatment, when, and under what conditions. Thus, the shortest, best, but perhaps not altogether satisfying answer to this question is that each person needs to make this decision by taking into account what they know about themselves, what their physical and psychological health risks are regardless of their weight, and what risks are associated with their weight. Then, with their primary care provider, mental healthcare provider, and possibly important loved ones, a well-informed decision can be made with respect to what form of treatment should be pursued, if any, and under what circumstances may it make sense to reverse course and either stop treatment altogether or pursue treatment to begin with. Knowing as much as possible about all forms of weight-loss treatment can help someone determine which forms they might consider and which they would not. Moreover, knowing as much about themselves as possible in terms of life goals that may or may not be affected by how much they weigh can also serve to help each person make an informed decision.

Social Stigma, Acceptance, and Prevention

34. What effect do anti-fat bias and discrimination have on the emotional health of an obese individual?

As noted in the answer to Question 7, anti-fat bias refers to a kind of prejudice that is focused on those who have fat bodies. This type of bias is also referred to as weight bias, weight stigma, and weight discrimination. If you are not familiar with what anti-fat bias might feel like or look like, it is, unfortunately, relatively easy to find examples of anti-fat bias via social media and other sources. Those with larger bodies are often the target of jokes and cruel comments. There is a great deal of research on the impact of this type of bias on the overall well-being of those who are the targets of this type of discrimination.

To give you an idea about how prevalent anti-fat bias can be and the effect it can have, a study called the *National Epidemiologic Survey on Alcohol and Related Conditions* asked more than 20,000 overweight and obese adults about the degree to which they perceived they have experienced weight discrimination. They were asked how common it was for them to actually be prevented from doing something because of their weight or the degree to which they felt like they could not do something because of their weight. This included things such as not getting adequate healthcare or health insurance, experiencing discrimination from their healthcare provider, and experiencing discrimination in public, at work, at school, or in any other setting or situation (see Question 35 for more information about how anti-fat bias affects healthcare). These same people were also asked about any psychological distress they have experienced, including mood and anxiety disorders, substance-use disorders, their degree of stress, and whether they have received any social support. Among those who stated they experienced weight-related discrimination, over half of them met the diagnostic criteria for at least one psychiatric disorder (e.g., a mood disorder, an anxiety disorder, an eating disorder, a substance-use disorder). The primary factor that seemed to contribute to the presence (or absence) of a psychiatric disorder was the degree to which they experienced stress. These researchers also found that having a good social support system did not necessarily protect these adults from the effects of perceived weight discrimination. Thus, when people believe they are being discriminated against because of their weight, they are highly likely to also experience a psychological disorder as a result of increased stress regardless of how much support they may have from friends and family.

Additional studies examining how anti-fat bias may impact overweight and obese individuals have reported similar findings to those of this national study. Some have suggested that weight stigma itself should be considered a public health issue such that those who experience weight stigma are likely to experience a decline in their overall health, including their psychological health. Some studies have found a connection between experiencing weight stigma and clinical depression, stating that weight stigma alone is a risk factor for developing this particular psychiatric disorder. Low self-esteem is often connected with clinical depression, and self-esteem levels have been shown to drop when weight-related discrimination is experienced. For those who might think that it is being overweight or obese that is the reason people might struggle psychologically, another study found this not to be the case. These researchers scientifically controlled for factors such as when someone became obese, how old they were, what their BMI was, and if they were male or female, and found that the increase in mental health issues could not be explained by any of these factors. The factor that did explain the presence of mental health issues, however, was weight stigma.

Although weight stigma and poor psychological well-being seem to be fairly well connected, the good news is that there are some things individuals can do to counteract this experience. When those who experience weight stigma use effective coping strategies to deal with it, they are less likely to subsequently experience distress or a drop in psychological well-being. Of course, not all coping strategies are universal, meaning that what works for one person may not work for another. So for one person, talking with a good friend about what they experienced may help to mitigate the negative impact of weight stigma, whereas for others, something like positive self-talk (i.e., saying positive things about yourself to yourself, such as "I am a good person") is an effective strategy. Additionally, in some cases, adopting an attitude of self-acceptance can be an effective coping strategy in the face of anti-fat bias. That is, accepting and appreciating yourself exactly as you are can be highly effective for many people to stave off the negative psychological effects of weight-based stigma. Ultimately, the idea is that when someone finds a strategy that works, it will likely continue to benefit them and can combat the deleterious effects of weight-based stigma.

35. How do anti-fat bias and discrimination affect the healthcare of obese individuals?

A substantial amount of research has been conducted examining the extent to which anti-fat bias among healthcare professionals affects the treatment and care of those who are obese or overweight. Anti-fat bias is decidedly a cultural phenomenon that can be seen in any situation in which a person who is overweight or obese finds themselves, and the healthcare setting is such a situation. Since obesity was recently officially declared a disease by the American Medical Association (see Question 43 for information about whether obesity should be considered a disease), healthcare providers have a greater incentive to intervene with those who have more pounds on their body than the BMI chart suggests they should (see Questions 1 and 2 for more information about BMI). Furthermore, since healthcare providers exist within a culture in which anti-fat bias is relatively commonplace and in which a war on obesity has been declared, it should not be surprising to learn that anti-fat bias can and does exist among healthcare professionals. Certainly not all healthcare professionals have an anti-fat bias (or its counterpart, the pro-thin bias), but when it does exist, it can have a negative impact on patients and their overall well-being.

Though it was not referred to as such several decades ago, anti-fat bias has existed among some healthcare professionals at least as far back as the 1960s. A study published in this era found a negative bias among healthcare professionals, with some physicians stating that they would rather not have an obese person as a patient, and if they did, they would expect that any health-related intervention would be a failure. Thus, this response seems to reflect an attitude of "Why bother? Whatever I recommend won't work anyway." Contemporary research has shown that anti-fat bias among healthcare professionals occurs at a rate lower than that found among the general population, but some healthcare professionals still have a bias against larger bodies that may extend to who the person is as a human being. That is, the bias includes thinking about fat people negatively in terms of personal characteristics such as intelligence (e.g., "fat people are stupid") or degree of motivation (e.g., "fat people are lazy"). Given these findings, some researchers have endeavored to figure out if healthcare providers in training can be taught to divest themselves of anti-fat bias or be prevented from developing it in the first place.

Studies examining anti-fat bias prevention efforts reported promising findings but did not reliably show that healthcare providers could be helped to develop a less-biased perspective. One study found that healthcare providers in training reduced the degree to which they explicitly stated they were biased against fat people, but other results indicated that the anti-fat bias still existed. The bias was simply not as obvious or was not a consciously held belief. These less conscious or unconsciously held beliefs are referred to as implicit biases and are believed by some researchers to be so deeply held that they are more resistant to change than the beliefs we are consciously aware of. Another group of researchers who examined the research on anti-fat bias among healthcare professionals found that changes can be made to their understanding of what causes obesity (i.e., that there are multiple factors, not all of which are under an individual's control; see Questions 9–19 for more information about causes and risk factors related to obesity); however, changing the prejudice or bias against those who are obese did not meaningfully occur. Knowing that anti-fat bias does exist in the healthcare professions and elsewhere, and that it can be resistant to change, it is also important to then examine what, if any, impact this bias can have on the overweight and obese patients these healthcare providers serve.

As noted in Question 34, experiencing anti-fat bias can negatively impact someone's psychological well-being and overall mental health. It can also negatively impact someone's physical health. Researchers have found that regular exposure to anti-fat bias has been connected to changes in a person's biochemistry involved with how body fat is accumulated and stored. It has also been associated with an increase in blood-sugar intolerance. Collectively, these findings mean that the more stress someone experiences as a result of anti-fat bias, the more their body will change how it metabolizes and stores food and its byproducts. These researchers took these findings a step further and noted that anti-fat bias may ultimately have the same negative effects on one's physical well-being as other pervasive forms of prejudice and discrimination, such as racism. Such negative effects have included different forms of cancer, high blood pressure, and other cardiovascular problems. Anti-fat bias among healthcare professionals may contribute to a worsening of well-being among those they are trying to treat. Anti-fat bias among healthcare professionals can also negatively impact the type of treatment they provide, which can further exacerbate existing health-related symptoms.

Healthcare providers who treat patients who are obese have been found to spend less time with such patients, to provide less health-related education, to be less likely to provide preventative care or diagnostic screenings (e.g., cancer screenings), or to advise larger-bodied patients on intervention or treatment methods other than weight loss. Moreover, when an overweight or obese patient seeks medical advice for existing symptoms, weight is often identified by the healthcare provider as the cause of whatever has brought the patient in to be seen. As noted previously in this answer, some healthcare providers view obese patients as lazy and as unlikely to follow treatment recommendations. This view can lead a healthcare provider to communicate less effectively overall and to spend less time with the patient to educate them about their health. One study, for example, found that among patients whose primary symptom was shortness of breath, obese patients were advised to make lifestyle changes while their normal-weight counterparts received medication.

In addition to anti-fat bias among healthcare professionals themselves, some clinics and offices are set up in such a way that they reflect an anti-fat bias. This can include waiting rooms that cannot safely and/or comfortably accommodate larger bodies (e.g., chairs are too narrow to sit in at all or without pain or discomfort), and medical equipment that cannot accommodate larger bodies (e.g., blood pressure cuffs that cannot fit around larger arms).

When patients are studied directly, obese patients have been found to feel embarrassed and humiliated when they experience anti-fat bias in a healthcare setting, which can further lead to a decrease in quality and quantity of care. When experiencing strong emotions, it can be difficult to concentrate and remember important information. Thus, patients who experience embarrassment and humiliation in response to healthcare settings with an anti-fat bias may not fully process what they are being told by their healthcare provider and may, therefore, misunderstand or not at all hear what is being said. Such an experience has also been found to result in obese patients' being less likely to schedule or keep appointments for routine checkups and other preventative screenings, thereby delaying diagnosis of an existing condition or having one go untreated.

For those that may be wondering about information indicating that higher healthcare costs are associated with obese patients, which would imply that obese individuals have greater healthcare needs (i.e., have more physical problems compared to those with "normal weight" bodies), critics note that what is not taken into consideration when making calculations about healthcare costs are the things noted above: not receiving preventative care at a rate similar to those who are not obese, focusing only on weight as the cause of a set of symptoms, and not receiving as much health-related education compared to those who are not obese. Thus, these critics indicate that any higher healthcare costs associated with those who are obese may have less to do with more health problems, per se, and more to do with delayed care or inadequate care that allows early-stage disease processes to advance to stages that are harder to treat. Others have noted that these higher costs may be a result of the patient's repeated but unsuccessful efforts to lose weight (advice they likely received from their healthcare provider; see questions 4 and 12 for more information about yo-yo dieting, also known as weight cycling).

Overall, obese individuals who have already experienced anti-fat bias with their current healthcare providers or fear they may experience it in a new practice are more likely to be reluctant to attend an appointment when they expect to encounter a negative attitude at best or discrimination at worst. Despite the fact that many healthcare providers treat all of their patients with kindness and respect if the patient is new to the practice or to a particular healthcare provider, the patient will not know what to expect. They may expect to receive substandard care yet again if they have experienced anti-fat bias in previous healthcare settings.

36. What effect do anti-fat bias and discrimination have on children's academic performance?

In comparison to what is known about the impact of anti-fat bias on a person's well-being in the healthcare setting (see Question 35 for more information), less is known about the degree to which children are adversely impacted in the school setting, particularly with respect to academic performance. Anti-fat bias among children has been demonstrated by age eight and may be present in preschoolers as early as age three. Research has also shown that typical, negative stereotypes regarding obesity (see Question 7 for more information about anti-fat bias) exists among children regardless of whether or not they are provided a medical explanation for another child's obesity. Thus, the reason as to why someone may be obese does not mitigate the negative beliefs about and attitudes toward those who are obese. These perceptions continue and become more conspicuous throughout the high school years and into college. Interestingly, the self-esteem levels of obese and nonobese children are roughly the same around age three, but once a child enters K–12 schooling, there is dramatic drop in self-esteem among those who are obese. This is especially true when an obese child holds the perception that they are to blame for their body shape and size (see Questions 9–19 for more information about causes and risk factors for obesity). Extensive research in this area makes clear the fact that obese children are likely to be bullied in schools and that being bullied because of one's appearance has a greater negative impact on girls compared to boys.

As was previously noted, there is not as much research in the area of anti-fat bias and its effect on a child's education in comparison to what is known about the effects of anti-fat bias in healthcare; however, the research that does exist in this area paints an unfortunate and potentially harmful picture. The studies that have been conducted show a pattern that obese children are more likely than their nonobese peers to miss more school, have more detentions, have a higher rate of tardiness, participate less in sports, and underperform.

The findings of such studies have led some researchers to conclude that efforts need to be made to help obese children participate in school more effectively and to attain regular and on-time attendance. Although this is not necessarily a bad approach to take, critics have noted that most of these studies did not examine the degree to which these children were exposed to anti-fat bias and discrimination, both of which may very well explain behaviors such as arriving late to school, not participating in activities, and skipping school altogether—many of these things, if they occur frequently enough, will result in detention and underperformance. Thus, the school-related factors found among obese children and adolescents may not be a function of obesity specifically but of the prejudice and discrimination to which they are exposed on a regular basis. As a result, some researchers and advocates have stated that rather than focusing on obese children, the focus should be intervention and prevention efforts targeting anti-fat bias and discrimination.

A recent study of teachers in K–12 schools found that most teachers connected obesity with lower academic achievement; however, the reasons these teachers made the connection were not due to what one might expect if the teachers harbored an anti-fat bias. The teachers did not believe obese students performed poorly because they were lazy or were not as smart; rather, they indicated that lower levels of confidence seemed to account for lower academic achievement. These teachers also noted that obese children were more likely to be the target of bullying, which they believed resulted in lower levels of self-esteem, which contributed to an overall tendency to withdraw. One study, however, did find that some adolescent females who were 50–60 pounds heavier than their peers had a grade point average (GPA) that was 8–10 percentile points lower. This finding did not hold for males and seemed only to affect white females. Although the reason for this difference is not known, the researcher speculated that there may be school (and work-related) discrimination against white females who are obese, which may further reflect the anti-fat–biased notion that obese white females have less to offer than any other demographic.

37. What effect do governmental programs and campaigns have on obesity?

Governmental fitness programs date back to the Dwight D. Eisenhower administration when the President's Council on Youth Fitness was established. Eventually this Council was renamed the President's Council on Sports, Fitness and Nutrition. Among the first initiatives implemented by the federal government to specifically address concerns about overweight and obese children and adolescents occurred in 1993. At this time a committee was convened for the purpose of providing recommendations for the assessment and treatment of overweight and obesity. The committee recommended that BMI should be used to determine which children were obese (see Questions 1 and 2 for more information about BMI). It was not until 1999, however, that the Centers for Disease Control and Prevention (CDC) began to take action on what was then called the obesity epidemic. This occurred following the publication of an article in the *Journal of the American Medical Association* (JAMA) that illustrated the increase in the rate of obesity in the United States. This was followed in 2000 by the release of CDC growth charts on which a child's height and weight have traditionally been tracked by a pediatrician; however, the 2000 version included tracking BMI for the first time. The year 2000 also saw the funding of several state-directed programs designed to address issues related to nutrition, physical activity, and obesity.

Since the year 2000, the CDC in partnership with other state, federal, and international organizations has developed other initiatives designed to improve the health of human beings, with the focus on reducing the rate of obesity and overweight. These initiatives provided recommendations for having healthier workplaces, breastfeeding, increasing physical activity among children, and increasing physical activity among older adults. In 2003 behavioral strategies for preventing overweight and obesity were released and included recommendations for the amount of fruits and vegetables that should be eaten in a day, how much physical activity should be engaged in, and how much screen time should be allowed. In 2008 the U.S. Department of Health and Human Services (DHHS) released the *2008 Physical Activity Guidelines for Americans*, which provided recommendations for optimal physical activity for children and adolescents, adults, older adults, pregnant women, adults with disabilities, and those with chronic medical conditions. The *Guidelines* also included recommendations for engaging in safe physical activity. In 2009 guidelines for healthy children included reducing the amount of sugary drinks children consume. In February 2010 then First Lady Michelle Obama introduced her childhood-obesity-prevention initiative called *Let's Move!* There have been myriad other governmental initiatives from 1999 to the present.

Data collected via the *National Health and Nutrition Examination Survey (NHANES)* showed a decrease in the rates of obesity among children aged two to five during the periods of 2003–2004 and 2011–2012. The rates of obesity among all other age groups showed that the rates had leveled off or reached a plateau. The *Pediatric Nutrition Surveillance System (PedNSS)* showed a similar trend among young children, indicating a decline in obesity among children aged two to four years and decreases in childhood obesity in six states. Credit for these aggregate findings is attributed, in part, to the increased awareness of the "obesity epidemic," starting with the article on the increasing rates of obesity published in 1999. From that point forward, government funding was directed toward addressing and staving off the obesity rate, and the general public, at the very least, became aware of others' concerns (e.g., government, health-care providers) about obesity. This growth in awareness may explain the fact that over half of the U.S. population believes that the most important health concern of the nation is childhood obesity. As a result, parents in particular have made changes to their own and their children's nutrition and physical-activity habits. This is evidenced, at least for improved nutrition, by data showing that those in the United States are consuming less fast food and fewer sugary drinks.

Though all of this sounds promising, those responsible for instituting many of the overweight- and obesity-prevention initiatives have expressed concern about whether or not these changes can be sustained in the long term. They have indicated that these efforts have taken a "top-down" approach, meaning that they have started at the top with the government, which has worked to get information and recommendations for behavioral changes to the states, local communities, individual health-care practitioners, and families. Critics point to the fact that other cultural changes, such as the civil rights movement, were "bottom-up" or grassroots initiatives. Those efforts started first with the people in their communities, and eventually their concerns made their way up to the federal government. Thus, some have indicated that in order for prevention and treatment efforts with respect to obesity to be sustained, they must take on a grassroots quality. Additionally, since many of the federal efforts in recent years were heavily endorsed by and/or initiated by the Obama administration, some have noted that future administrations may not be as committed to addressing the issue and that it will, therefore, take a back seat to whatever that particular administration views as important. Finally, some have noted that the term *obesity* can be used in a derogatory way. Since the term *obesity* is not merely a descriptor of one's body weight but has a great deal of negativity associated with it, some researchers have speculated that this might explain why the general public has been shown to be unlikely to recognize when they or their children are obese—which can further mean that some people are less likely to take seriously any efforts to address obesity. Therefore, it has been recommended that a shift occur away from obesity specifically and toward something like "wellness," which would not only encompass nutrition and physical activity but would also include other factors associated with overall well-being such as mental health.

The long-term sustainability of current prevention programs also requires that those involved communicate effectively across agencies or constituencies so that efforts to increase physical activity, increase the intake of fruits and vegetables, and decrease the intake of sugary drinks have a common overall agenda (e.g., wellness) and are mutually beneficial. For example, the market for sugary drinks is significant (in 2010 the dollar amount spent was over $14 billion), and there, predictably, has been strong opposition to governmental policies that may interfere with the continued purchase of such drinks. Finally, recent research has noted that the cost-effectiveness of any intervention must be evaluated. This means that while some obesity-prevention efforts may or may not show results, it is important to include how much it costs someone or a health-care agency (financially) to lower BMI and whether or not that intervention was cost effective and therefore "worth it."

38. What responsibility do public services have to accommodate people who are obese?

Public services refer to any business that supplies a product such as electricity or water and services provided for the public interest such as healthcare facilities, air travel, or restaurants. These services may be privately owned or maintained by a governmental agency (i.e., city/town, state, or federal). The issue of the degree to which public services should be responsible for accommodating people of size is a matter of debate that is often heated. The debate often occurs between those who think public services should accommodate people of all shapes and sizes because not doing so contributes to a decline in the well-being among those who are not accommodated, those who believe such accommodation may translate to higher costs for all people who access those services, and those who believe that accommodating larger body sizes encourages an unhealthy lifestyle.

One service industry that seems to be a lightning rod for this debate is the airline industry. One group of researchers posed the question: Whose responsibility is it to be sure larger bodies have an appropriate place on an airplane, the persons themselves or the airlines? These same researchers found that although overweight or obese passengers had plenty to say about what it is like to fly as someone with a larger body, those who were not overweight or obese seemed to have even more to say about the issue. These passengers noted that they felt "disgusted" by having to sit next to an obese passenger, that their rights were violated if the larger person's body "invaded" their space, that there might be an issue of safety particularly in an emergency, and that they wondered about subsidizing larger passengers because of their increased weight, citing the fact that if they have to pay more for a heavier piece of luggage, then larger passengers should have to pay more too. In fact, some airlines do require larger passengers to purchase two seats. This is done not necessarily because of weight, per se (although that is likely a factor), but because the body size takes up more space than a typical airline seat provides. As of 2012, the vast majority of airline companies did not have an explicit policy with regard to what to do if a passenger's body was too large to fit in a standard seat. Airlines that did had policies that ranged from requiring the passenger to purchase an extra seat to not allowing them to board the plane if they had not purchased an extra seat and there were no additional seats available. Although clear policies related to accommodating various body sizes would likely help streamline ticket purchases and boarding procedures, these researchers noted that since larger-bodied passengers are explicitly singled out, these policies may inadvertently justify bad and potentially discriminatory behavior on the part of fellow passengers and crew members. These researchers indicated that all data suggest that the average body size is projected to get larger rather than smaller, and it would behoove the industry to take note and change the size of its seats to accommodate a greater diversity of body sizes.

Fitness and exercise facilities constitute another service industry that is patronized by people of myriad body shapes and sizes. Regular exercise has benefits for everyone regardless of body size, and, of course, those who are overweight or obese are usually strongly encouraged to exercise for the explicit purpose of losing weight; however, they are often met with negativity when they do exercise. Overweight and obese exercisers have reported that they are ridiculed based on their body size, they are ridiculed for engaging in exercise while having a large body, they are ridiculed for wearing the same type of clothing that their smaller-sized counterparts wear during exercise, and they are ridiculed for moving their body in ways similar to their smaller-sized counterparts when engaged in exercise. When this is the experience of an exerciser who is overweight or obese, the result can be that they stop exercising in public or altogether regardless of whether or not anyone can see them. Researchers have found that an anti-fat bias (see Question 7 for more information about this bias) can be held by fellow exercisers and fitness professionals, and that exercisers who had never been overweight or obese had a stronger anti-fat bias compared to those who had previously had a larger body. Consequently, researchers have recommended that fitness and exercise facilities should, at minimum, train their professionals to better understand the nature of obesity so that they can more effectively and positively interact with their larger-bodied patrons.

In terms of other services for which body size may be an issue (e.g., restaurants, educational settings), there is little incentive other than an owner's or manager's personal choice to be sure all body sizes are accommodated. Obesity itself is not a protected class in terms of discrimination. That is, discrimination laws that exist usually identify certain classes or groups of people against whom discrimination is a punishable offense. These include groups based on race or ethnicity, religion, sexual orientation, and so on. Despite the fact that obesity is not identified as a protected class, some individuals have successfully and others unsuccessfully sued various public services primarily for inadequate accommodation with respect to seating.

39. What effect do weight-loss–related television reality shows have on obesity?

Weight-loss television shows range from those that are purely information-based to those that are entertainment-type reality series. Over the years, weight-loss–related shows have included *The Biggest Loser*, *Extreme Weight Loss*, *The Dr. Oz Show*, *Celebrity Fat Fighters*, *My Diet Is Better Than Yours*, *Obese: A Year to Save My Life* (an *Extreme Makeover* show), *Celebrity Fit Club*, *Cold Turkey*, *Honey*, *We're Killing the Kids*, *Weighing In*, and *Fat March*. Some of these shows lasted only one year or were planned for one episode, whereas others were on air for several years—the longest of which was *The Biggest Loser*. The intent of these shows is typically to inspire people to lose weight ostensibly to improve their health. However, concern among some healthcare providers has led them to question whether or not such shows truly have a beneficial impact not only on the participants themselves but also on those who watch the shows. The concern was strong enough that researchers have taken to studying the impact these shows actually have. Most of the research that has been conducted examined the impact of *The Biggest Loser*, which aired from 2004 to 2016.

Television viewers of *The Biggest Loser* numbered close to 10 million, and it was considered to be among the most popular reality televisions shows in the United States. The show's popularity meant that it was franchised to a multitude of other countries. The premise of the show was to cast overweight or obese contestants, both male and female, who would compete for money by losing the most weight (based on the percentage of body weight lost). The contestants worked with trainers who were responsible for designing workout and nutrition plans. Critiques of the show alleged that the show was dangerous due to the encouragement of rapid weight loss, the potential malnourishment or dehydration of contestants, their overexertion, and the possibility that some contestants were given or took weight-loss pills to facilitate weight loss.

Some researchers found that the show could appropriately be considered irresponsible because it promoted weight-loss efforts that are typically unrealistic (some contestants lost 100 pounds in three months) and unsustainable (there are reports of many contestants regaining all of the weight they lost plus more). Moreover, researchers have indicated that the show perpetuated the notion that weight loss and obesity specifically are within an individual's control and that, therefore, those who are obese have only themselves to blame (see Question 19 for more information about obesity and willpower and Questions 9–18 for information about causes and risk factors). This can lead to a biased perception of overweight and obese individuals and can perpetuate anti-fat bias and discrimination (see Questions 7 and 34–38 for more information about anti-fat bias and its effects).

Researchers also found that those who were preoccupied with their own body weight and shape were more likely to watch a show like *The Biggest Loser* and that this type of preoccupation is known to be a risk factor for eating disorders, which have the highest mortality rate of any psychiatric illness. Additionally, some researchers concluded that the show was full of so much misinformation that those who were most negatively impacted were the viewers who did not question whether or not what they saw on the show was accurate and/or healthy.

Other researchers examined whether the show truly resulted in healthy behavior change for those who watched the show. Findings indicate that while viewers might have experienced some degree of inspiration as they watched contestants dramatically change their bodies, and in some cases their views of themselves and others, it rarely translated into the engagement of health-related behaviors in viewers.

Finally, another group of scholars examined not only how shows like *The Biggest Loser* impact individuals and their perceptions of how weight loss works (e.g., whether or not it is within the individual's control) but also how exposure to such shows impacts the work healthcare practitioners can and cannot do with patients who watch the shows. They noted, as others have, that *The Biggest Loser*'s strong and consistent message that weight loss is well within an individual's control—they just have to try hard enough—means that any efforts to educate these patients that body shape and size are contingent on a complex interaction of factors (see Questions 9–19 for causes and risk factors associated with obesity) may not be fully heard or taken in by the patient. That is, viewers of the show may be so convinced that their body weight and shape are entirely their "fault" that they are not likely to consider factors such as genetics, their access to and ability to afford healthier foods, and so on. The message of this and other similar shows is, therefore, believed to be at odds with efforts to address more societally based and global issues such as food availability and access to safe spaces for exercise. Therefore, it has been recommended by some that shows such as *The Biggest Loser* ought not to be used as celebratory examples of what is possible but as examples of something that interferes with our ability to engage in healthy behaviors and interferes with our ability to treat others with respect and dignity.

Ultimately, those who have researched the effects of *The Biggest Loser* have found that it may, in fact, perpetuate weight-related stigma, which the show was designed, in part, to prevent.

40. How are schools addressing obesity and the bullying of obese children?

Bullying in schools is not a new phenomenon, nor is weight-related bullying. However, in recent years schools have recognized the need to actively address bullying that occurs for any reason, and weight-related bullying specifically. Students, parents, and teachers all seem to agree that kids are more likely to be bullied for their weight than for any other reason. This is not to suggest that bullying for other reasons does not occur nor is any less important to address, simply that weight is likely to be the most common reason.

Researchers have found that children and adolescents who are overweight or obese show psychosocial impairment that can last for years. The findings are particularly strong for overweight or obese girls. In general, researchers reported that the higher a child's BMI when overweight or obese, the lower their level of self-esteem, the higher the degree of body dissatisfaction, and the more symptoms related to an eating disorder are reported. All of these may persist during their developmentally formative years (i.e., childhood and adolescence).

With respect to bullying, overweight or obese girls were more likely to be bullied than their overweight or obese male counterparts; however, both sexes reported more bullying than their normal-weight peers. Much of the research that uncovers psychosocial impairment (e.g., low self-esteem, high body dissatisfaction) among those who are overweight or obese indicates that this can be explained in terms of whether or not a child has been or is being bullied. That is, overweight and obese children are likely to suffer a great deal less (if at all) when weight-related bullying does not occur. Some researchers have concluded that children and adolescents who develop eating disorders may do so in part because they had been bullied because of their weight.

As of 2016 only three states, New York, New Hampshire, and Maine, had anti-bullying laws that explicitly included weight-related bullying or bullying based on physical appearance. Those who influence policy makers have suggested that issues related to weight-based bullying should be included in health-related curricula, and that there should be requirements for teachers and coaches to receive adequate education with regard to preventing and identifying weight-related bullying. They have also suggested that physical education programs should be modified to be more inclusive and supportive of children with larger bodies. Finally, they strongly suggest that anti-bullying policies need to be improved in schools and that more laws need to be in place designed to protect overweight or obese students.

Interestingly, some research has indicated that the degree to which people believed obesity is the result of poor choices or poor willpower (see Question 19 for more information about willpower and obesity) affected the degree to which they believed schools or the government should be involved in policy making regarding weight-related bullying. For example, those who do not think the individual is to blame for being obese were more likely to believe that schools and the government should take action to address weight-related bullying. Additionally, those who believed that the degree of willpower did not factor into whether or not someone is obese believed both schools and the government should be actively involved in weight-related anti-bullying efforts. When research participants reported that they knew someone who had been the target of weight-related bullying, they agreed that schools and the government should take action; however, those who were on the receiving end of the bullying did not endorse school or government involvement in weight-related anti-bullying efforts.

When inquiring with educators, specifically, regarding their opinions about weight-related bullying and how schools handle this issue, educators seemed to overwhelmingly agree that schools should have policies in place that help to prevent weight-related bullying, and that help to protect students who are the targets of such bullying. Educators specifically supported school-based efforts that promote awareness of weight-related bullying and that shield students from being bullied about their weight to begin with. Researchers have concluded that given the resources directed toward nutrition in schools and wellness-related policies, implementing anti-bullying policies should not be too difficult.

Educators tended to agree with the general population that school is not the place to assess and/or track the height and weight of students. So called "BMI Report Cards" have been incorporated into many school systems throughout the United States; however, many states no longer require them due, in part, to public concern about the impact of such report cards on the well-being of children, including making overweight and obese children targets for bullies, and due also to the finding that these report cards have been shown in some research to have negative effects on children, including the development of an eating disorder.

When initiating weight-related bullying–prevention programs in schools, educators agreed that a multidisciplinary approach is warranted. Many teachers indicated that not only should teachers be involved in the development of weight-related anti-bullying efforts, but so should school counselors, school administrators, coaches, school nurses, parents, and the students themselves. Researchers have suggested that healthcare providers outside of the school setting should also be involved in weight-related anti-bullying efforts, particularly when students are experiencing bullying by teachers and/or family members.

When intervention programs are in place, they can be categorized based on whether the interventions are schoolwide or targeted. School-wide interventions focus on all students, students' parents or primary caregivers, and all school personnel. Targeted interventions focus on a small subset of the school population such as the bullies themselves or those who are the targets of bullying. Much of the research on school-based anti-bullying interventions is on bullying in general and not specifically on weight-based bullying. One group of researchers who summarized what is known about anti-bullying efforts in schools indicated that the research shows most programs do not work. They concluded this may be due, in part, to flaws inherent in how these programs were studied; however, in addition to ensuring that anti-bullying programs are effectively studied, researchers have identified a number of other factors that may make current and future anti-bullying efforts (whether for weight-related bullying or bullying for other reasons) more effective. They also noted that the original schoolwide anti-bullying program that most programs are modeled after, the Olweus Bullying Prevention Program (OBPP), was developed in the early 1990s and implemented in Norway where there was high buy-in by school personnel who were also well trained, and class sizes were small. Schools in the United States, for example, can be larger than those in Norway, but perhaps most importantly, many teachers in the United States balk against schoolwide programs because they do not feel that they have time to incorporate the program in an already tight curriculum and/or they believe that bullying should be addressed in the home by parents or primary caregivers.

A more recent schoolwide program developed in Finland called KiVa (an acronym for a Finnish phrase that translates to "against bullying") has shown more promise. This program focuses its efforts on bystanders to bullying (i.e., those who are not bullying nor who are the targets of bullying but who witness bullying). The focus is on helping bystanders feel more empathy for victims and encouraging them to help victims when they are being bullied. A program developed in Canada called Walk

Away, Ignore, Talk It Out, Seek Help (WITS) was designed for elementary school students in first through third grades to help them develop the skills they need to effectively resolve interpersonal problems. Both KiVa and WITS have shown effectiveness in their respective countries, but neither has been studied in the United States. One program that was developed in the United States called Steps to Respect was designed for elementary school students and has its focus on aggression that occurs in relationships in the form of gossip or ostracism. All three of these schoolwide interventions are believed to represent interventions that can be considered well-designed and provide a solid basis for prevention efforts.

Targeted interventions can focus on bullies or victims. The most well-known and studied forms of intervention focus on how bullies think and behave, particularly in situations in which it is unclear what is going on. Kids who are aggressive, who are also often bullies, tend to assume that their peers are intentionally behaving in a hostile manner to them even when it is unclear whether or not a particular behavior was intended. Accidently bumping into such a kid in the hallway, for example, is likely to be interpreted by an aggressive kid as an intentional act, and, therefore, they have to decide if they are going to "retaliate" or not. A program developed and implemented in the United States in the early 1990s called Fast Track focuses on helping kids at risk for being aggressive and ultimately a bully learn how to accurately interpret social interactions, effectively solve interpersonal problems, understand emotions, engage in effective communication, and develop self-control. This program also includes training for parents, and elements of the program were continued and individualized with the children throughout tenth grade. Results indicate that the most at-risk kids for aggression and bullying, particularly boys, showed fewer incidences of aggression and bullying even after the program ended. Currently, effective programs that help victims change their own social cognitive processes (i.e., how they think about and interpret their interactions with peers) do not seem to exist. Since victims of bullying tend to blame themselves for being bullied to begin with, researchers indicate that victims also need assistance with changing how they think about their interactions with others, particularly with bullies.

Researchers and program developers note that whether programs are schoolwide or targeted they must take into account the fact that times of transition can make at-risk students more vulnerable to bullying and its effects. They suggest that programs should ensure support services are in place for those who may struggle with, for example, transitioning from grade school to middle school or middle school to high school. Of particular importance is the benefit of having friendships. At-risk students who can count at least one peer as their friend tend to fare better than those who feel completely disconnected from their peers. Another identified point of focus is on incorporating efforts to address more covert forms of bullying, such as social ostracism or bullying that takes place online (i.e., cyberbullying). Most current programs focus on more obvious forms of bullying such as physical and verbal aggression but fail to take into account what may be less obvious but equally harmful forms of bullying. Additionally, the nature of child and adolescent peer groups and the social hierarchy that exists result in some individual students or groups of students being more powerful than others. Researchers indicate that anti-bullying campaigns need to find ways to involve and thereby use the influence of these students to help promote prosocial interactions with all students.

41. Does pursuing the culturally expected body type affect obesity?

The culturally expected body types in western cultures are the thin-ideal for women and the muscular-ideal for men (see Question 6 for more information about these ideals). Briefly, the thin-ideal for women is the expectation that in order to be attractive, women should be thin, with low body fat, but also have some curves, whereas the muscular-ideal for men is the expectation that in order to be attractive, men need to have well-developed and well-defined muscles with low body fat. For either sex, the respective ideal is naturally achieved for a very small percentage of the population (i.e., well below 5 percent). Thus, in order for the remaining percentage of the population to achieve either ideal, males and females must engage in varying degrees of weight loss and/or exercise in order to drop weight and/or reduce body fat.

Most of those who engage in weight-loss efforts, which may or may not involve starting or ramping up exercise efforts, will find that they are unable to sustain what they are doing for very long. This is more likely to be the case when calorie intake is restricted to an amount per day that is well below what the body needs in order to function adequately and/or if they are engaged in an exercise routine that they do not enjoy for any reason. When an individual gets to the point that they "can't take it anymore" and are tired of not eating enough or not eating foods they had eliminated from their intake, or they cannot face exercising any longer, they will likely resume what they had been doing prior to their new weight-loss routine—eating a lot more and a greater variety of foods and exercising a lot less or not at all. The result is predictable: they will gain the weight back plus additional pounds. This can often lead to a pattern of weight cycling or yo-yo dieting that ultimately results in weighing more than they did before they started losing weight the first time, and can result in significant health issues (see Questions 4 and 12 for more information about yo-yo dieting). It is often the case that there is a history of yo-yo dieting for those who are trying to lose weight "for good." For a smaller percentage of those who pursue the thin- or muscular-ideal, the result of such efforts can trigger the development of a serious and potentially fatal mental health issue: eating disorders.

Eating disorders have the highest mortality rate of any psychiatric illness, with the most common causes of death being cardiac arrest or dying by suicide, particularly among those diagnosed with anorexia nervosa. A percentage of those who are susceptible to developing an eating disorder (the current understanding of eating disorders is that genetic factors interact with environmental factors, which explains why some people develop an eating disorder and others do not) will develop anorexia nervosa, some will develop bulimia nervosa, others will develop binge eating disorder (BED), and some may experience more than one eating disorder. It is not possible at this time to predict which eating disorder(s), if any, will develop for any particular person.

With regard to how eating disorders interact with obesity, some people mistakenly assume that binge eating disorder and obesity go hand in hand or even that they are one and the same. Both accounts are inaccurate. As noted in misconception number 2 in this book, not everyone who is obese has binge eating disorder, and not everyone who has binge eating disorder is obese. This may seem counterintuitive; however, when one considers all factors that account for one's body shape and size (see Questions 9–19 for more information about causes and risk factors for obesity), it becomes clear that while binging in and of itself is likely to cause weight gain, it is not necessarily going to result in a BMI measurement that classifies someone's body as obese (see Questions 1 and 2 for more information about BMI).

With respect to the other two eating disorders, anorexia nervosa and bulimia nervosa, the association with obesity is better understood as the individual being terrified that they will become fat or that they desperately want to no longer be fat. For anorexia nervosa specifically, the fear of gaining weight or becoming fat is one part of the diagnostic criteria. That is, those who are diagnosed with this disorder make decisions about food and exercise based on an intense fear (e.g., feeling terrified) of becoming fat. Thus, they severely restrict how much food they eat and often, though not always, engage in excessive exercise. Some individuals who have either diagnosis (anorexia nervosa or bulimia nervosa) may have a history of being overweight or obese. Some may intend to lose only a few pounds but find that they are then driven to try to lose more. Those who are diagnosed with bulimia nervosa will have a pattern of binge eating and purging (i.e., self-induced vomiting) or other compensatory behavior (e.g., using laxatives, fasting, excessive exercise) intended to "counteract" or get rid of the calories consumed during the binge, which is usually measured in terms of consuming thousands of calories at one time.

42. What effect do "love your body" campaigns have on obesity?

Love your body campaigns are any campaigns designed to provide tools to fight against the cultural standards for beauty and attractiveness (see Questions 6 and 41 for more information about the thin-ideal and the muscular-ideal) and to empower women and men to love their bodies as they are. Another term for these types of campaigns is body positivity. Body positivity began in the late 1960s and emerged from the fat acceptance movement. Most campaigns, however, do target women, though the messages in these campaigns are often transferable to men.

There are a number of campaigns designed to empower women to love their bodies as they are. The Love Your Body campaign was started by the National Organization for Women (NOW), which initiated the campaign to help women resist societal pressures to look a certain way. They have declared one day in October to be National Love Your Body Day (in 2017 that date was Wednesday, October 18).

In 2012 the hashtag #Fatkini was started by Gabi Fresh in collaboration with xoJane. This campaign encouraged women of size to take pictures of themselves in their bathing suits and post them to social media with the #Fatkini hashtag. In 2014 The Perfect Body campaign was started by Victoria's Secret. The campaign itself, however, featured only thin women. Amidst strong backlash, Victoria's Secret changed the campaign to A Body for Every Body but did not change the models representing the campaign. Curvy Kate Lingerie and the Dear Kate lingerie company recreated the Body for Every Body campaign but with body shape and size diversity.

The #ImNoAngel campaign was initiated by Lane Bryant and seemed to take aim at Victoria's Secret's penchant for showing only thin, curvy models. The #ImNoAngel campaign encouraged women of all sizes to post pictures of themselves to social media with the hashtag along with a "personal statement of confidence." The initial image published by Lane Bryant did feature larger-sized women but all of whom were seemingly similar in size. Thus, they received some criticism for not showing greater size diversity. The #ImNoModelEither campaign was started by Amanda Richards in response to Lane Bryant's #ImNoAngel campaign. She indicated that she did not see true size diversity in their campaign and, therefore, started a campaign for real women who did not represent the perfected look found among models of any size. She stated that campaigns like Lane Bryant's showcase "acceptable" plus-size women rather than women that more inclusively represent the plus-size community.

The Dove Campaign for Real Beauty (also known as the Dove Self-Esteem Project) is perhaps the most widely distributed and most familiar campaign. The campaign has been in place for over 10 years and has included videos and advertisements aimed at celebrating women of all shapes and sizes. Dove, as part of this campaign, has also conducted research on issues related to body image. A recent part of the campaign included initiating the hashtag #speakbeautiful designed to encourage positive self-talk about our bodies.

The Lose Hate, Not Weight campaign was started by Virgie Tovar, a fat activist, who intended to change the "not good enough" mindset that many people have about their bodies to a mindset of self-care and self-love. The What's Underneath Project initiated by Style Like U was designed to help people see their bodies in a nonobjectifying way. They had women talk about their thoughts and feelings about their bodies while getting undressed.

The LessIsMore campaign was started by a woman with a history of an eating disorder. Erin Treloar urged the fashion industry to reduce their use of Photoshop to "perfect" print images. She also founded RAW Beauty Talks for the purpose of helping girls feel confident in the bodies they have. The #Fatshion campaign does not seem to have a founder but rather seemed to grown naturally via social media. The hashtag is used by women of size who post photos of themselves and their outfits, thereby simultaneously celebrating fashion and large bodies.

Other corporate initiatives have included JCPenney's #HereIAm campaign, Aerie's #AierieReal, Dove's #MyBeautyMySay, and Ashley Stewart's Love Your Curves. Other social-media hashtags intended to celebrate body diversity have included #EffYourBeautyStandards, #HonorMyCurves, and #CelebrateMySize.

All of these campaigns are designed to celebrate the diversity of women's bodies and to help women love and accept their bodies as they are. The question remains: Are they having the intended effect?

Some critics have taken aim at corporate campaigns (e.g., Dove's Love Your Body campaign) that have capitalized on women's insecurities about their bodies, and rather than identifying what contributes to this problem (e.g., the beauty industry) or offering a solution to the problem, the companies simply produce advertisements and other media acknowledging that women feel bad about their bodies while promoting the notion that women of all sizes should be celebrated. Critics indicate that the ultimate message (though perhaps not intended) is that women have allowed themselves to feel bad about their bodies, and, therefore, it is women who need to make a change. Thus, critics indicate that the body positivity movement of the 1960s has changed from a subversive movement to one designed to sell you a product to help your feel better about yourself but one that ultimately benefits only the corporations profiting from poor body image among women.

Other critics have indicated that while the sentiment surrounding love your body campaigns is nice, it is simply surface-level encouragement that does not get at deeper issues that keep women from truly loving who they are and what their bodies look like. They indicate that for too long girls and women have been told that thin is not only superior to other body sizes, it comes with other perks such as getting the job you want, being happier, wearing cute clothing, having a desirable dating partner, and so on. That is, getting skinnier equals a better, happier life. Thus, it is not as simple as loving one's body if you don't think good things will happen to you, particularly if you have the "wrong" body shape and size.

Still others have indicated that love your body campaigns may be substituting one body ideal for another. Some have expressed concern over the idea that thin bodies may become as maligned as larger bodies have. This can leave consumers thinking that thin is not okay but that larger is. So what does that mean for those who are naturally thin? That they should no longer love their bodies and do everything they can to make their bodies larger? These critics suggest that those who struggle to love their bodies as they are should not attempt to suddenly love them but, rather, to learn to no longer judge their bodies or to at least become aware of how they think and feel about their bodies without trying to make themselves think and feel differently. By becoming more aware of what's going on in our hearts and minds, we can then become aware of how these thoughts and feelings affect our lives and how they may prevent us from having the life we want. Thus, such critics of love your body campaigns advocate for body acceptance rather than body love.

There has not been much formal research on the effectiveness of love your body campaigns. Some researchers who have examined popular love your body campaigns have identified several problems with such campaigns that seem to reflect what nonresearchers have noticed. These scientists have stated that what is problematic with these campaigns involves several things including the idea that many corporate campaigns espousing the "love your body" ideal, while talking about "natural" and "real" women, continue to use makeup and technology to ensure their models are attractive enough. Related to this is the notion that while the definition of beauty and attractiveness may have expanded, it has done so in only a small way. Models, whether professional or "real" women, are still expected to look good and not be or appear to be too fat. Researchers have also noted the paradox that many corporate love your body campaigns seem simultaneously invested in ensuring that women remain dissatisfied with their bodies, which will result in women's buying whatever product they are selling. Accompanying all of this is the idea that these campaigns seem to perpetuate the notion that if women hate their bodies, it is their responsibility to change them, as if women's body-esteem and self-esteem develop in a vacuum. Finally, researchers have noted that love your body campaigns have not only placed the responsibility of loving one's body squarely on the shoulders of women, they have also found another way to control women by indicating that they are not good enough unless they love their bodies, thus leaving women with yet another standard to live up to.

43. Should obesity be considered a disease?

Obesity has been seen as something to be treated, and thus "cured," since at least the time of the ancient Greeks. Consuming foods that are supposed to make you thin, taking amphetamines, going on low-calorie diets, and other "treatment" methods have been used and prescribed by medical personnel in an effort to help fat people become thin. And it was, and still is, believed that thinner automatically means healthier, although contemporary medical personnel recognize that thinness in the form of anorexia nervosa is not healthier. As a result, in 2014 the American Medical Association (AMA) officially declared obesity a disease.

Prior to the AMA's decision regarding obesity, the leadership in the organization tasked its Council on Science and Public Health (hereafter referred to as the Council) to explore whether or not obesity should be classified as a disease rather than continuing to refer to it as a "complex disorder," an "urgent chronic condition," an "epidemic," a "major health concern," or a "major public health problem." The Council examined information related to how the term *disease* is defined, how obesity is defined, whether or not BMI is an adequate measure for this purpose, and whether or not classifying obesity as a disease would result in improved health outcomes. Given the final decision of the AMA's membership to classify obesity as a disease, it may surprise some to know that the Council's conclusion was that "it is difficult to determine conclusively whether or not obesity is a medical disease state."

The Council reported that BMI itself is not an adequate measure to be used in clinical practice (i.e., in your doctor's office; see Questions 1 and 2 for more information about BMI). The Council stated that BMI is known to be an imperfect measure of body fat by the World Health Organization (WHO) and the National Heart, Lung, and Blood Institute (NHLBI) but is used because it is a relatively inexpensive screening tool used to predict disease risk. Ideally, BMI is used in conjunction with measures of blood pressure and blood lipids (i.e., fatty acid and cholesterol), which would provide a more comprehensive (and potentially accurate) picture of one's overall health. The Council goes on to note that BMI is not a good tool for identifying illness or disease risk for those with lower BMIs (i.e., BMI less than 30). They note that some people with lower BMIs may have excess body fat, a high degree of inflammation (which is associated with many disease processes), and metabolic symptoms typically associated with other disease processes that are usually associated with obesity (see Question 5 for more information about metabolic syndrome). By contrast, the Council acknowledged that those with a BMI above 30 do not necessarily have a high body-fat percentage, and even when they do they may not have other symptoms typically found in medical problems that are associated with obesity (e.g., high blood pressure, high lipid levels). What confounds that which is known about the inadequacy of BMI as a measure of health is that many studies have found that a high BMI is consistently associated with many diseases such as diabetes, sleep apnea, some forms of cancer, heart disease, stroke, and osteoarthritis, among others, thus leading many to believe that BMI is an effective measure of one's health status. When more closely examining the data on BMI, it can be seen that a high BMI is associated with but not necessarily a cause of the diseases linked to obesity, thus bolstering the notion that BMI is an inadequate measure of an individual's health status. Moreover, in support of their statement that BMI is an inadequate measure of health, the Council recognized the increasing number of studies reporting that a BMI in the overweight or lower obesity categories may actually help to prolong someone's life. That is, having a weight above the "normal" range on the BMI scale has been reported to be associated with a lower mortality risk.

With regard to how the term *disease* itself is defined, the Council reported that there is no one agreed-upon definition of *disease* and that the use of some definitions of *disease* would exclude things such as stroke, diabetes, alcoholism, and some psychiatric disorders from being classified as diseases. Furthermore, the Council noted that at any point in time the concept and definition of *disease* are affected by historical context and culture as well as changes based on what is discovered though scientific research. Consequently, the Council turned its attention to the notion of whether or not classifying obesity as a disease would be beneficial for people who are obese. They found support for the conflicting perspectives that it would be both potentially beneficial and potentially harmful to call obesity a disease.

The Council reported that in favor of classifying obesity as a disease, insofar as that classification would have a beneficial outcome for individuals, when something is declared a disease, governmental and private agencies are likely to direct financial and other resources to the study, prevention, and treatment of the disease in question. Moreover, if obesity were identified as a disease, the Food and Drug Administration (FDA) would be inclined to approve more medications designed to treat obesity—which ultimately means treating obesity via weight loss rather than treating any underlying processes such as those associated with metabolic syndrome (see Question 5 for more information about metabolic syndrome). Formally identifying obesity as a disease may also mean that more public policy and prevention programs will be developed to address obesity (see Question 37 for more information about governmental obesity programs and campaigns). Furthermore, if obesity were labeled a disease, there may be a reduction in stigma associated with elevated body weight and size as the general public learns that obesity is not something an individual can control and is not the result of laziness and lack of self-control (see Question 19 for information about obesity and willpower).

On the "labeling obesity as a disease will not be beneficial" side of the argument, the Council noted that recognizing obesity as a disease may mean that more resources are directed to surgical interventions (see Questions 31–33 for more information about bariatric surgery) and that patients and their medical providers may rely more on pharmaceuticals (see Questions 29 and 30 for more information about weight-loss medications) and surgical interventions, both of which can be expensive, as a means to change a patient's body size rather than focusing on helping patients develop healthy behaviors. They also noted that since BMI is still the measurement of choice, some people whose BMI is higher than 30 may be treated for a problem they don't have. That is, they may have a higher than "normal" BMI but do not have metabolic syndrome and thus are healthy in this regard. Moreover, those engaged in healthy behaviors (i.e., eating healthy and exercising) but do not lose any or enough weight to move them to a lower BMI category would still be considered as having a disease and would be encouraged if not pressured to seek medical intervention to treat their obese status. With respect to public policy that may be developed to combat obesity, the Council warned that such a focus may detract from other efforts to promote healthy living regardless of body shape or size, which they note could be detrimental to the health of everyone. Having obesity identified as a disease may also affect hiring practices, place an emphasis in employee health programs on weight rather than healthy behaviors, and raise health-insurance premiums. Finally, the Council noted that changing the status of obesity to that of a disease may mean for some that since they have a disease, they do not need to focus on engaging in healthy behaviors because having a disease is not something they can control, and labeling someone with a high enough BMI as being diseased may serve to alienate others, particularly if the focus is on making their body smaller rather than encouraging healthy behaviors.

After knowing some of the salient points found in the Council's report, it may make more sense as to why they concluded that classifying obesity as a disease is not clear cut, not only in terms of whether or not it fits the definition of disease, how it should be measured, and whether or not BMI truly reflects someone's health, but also in terms of whether or not labeling obesity as a disease is actually beneficial. Some researchers have examined whether or not the AMA's final decision to label obesity as a disease was the right decision to make.

One group of researchers found that while labeling obesity as a disease helped to decrease body dissatisfaction, they also found that those who were made aware that obesity was labeled as a disease made less healthy food choices than they had been making prior to learning about this label. Thus, the disease label likely made people think they had no control over their weight, so there was no reason to engage in efforts that might change their weight—which ultimately means, regardless of weight loss, that they were less likely to engage in behaviors that would promote their health and well-being. Researchers indicated that when patients are provided with disease-based information rather than public, health-based messages, there appeared to be less concern for health-focused choices; therefore, the type of message an obese individual received predicted the type of food choices they made.

❖

Case Studies

CASE 1: JESSICA

Jessica is a 12-year-old middle school student who has struggled with her weight as far back as she can remember. Her mother described her as a "happy, chubby baby who never lost her baby fat" but has reassured Jessica that once she goes through puberty, she will no longer be overweight. Jessica has already entered puberty and has found that she is only getting larger in places she'd rather not see expand. She believes her mother has lied to her, along with everyone else who tells her that they like her or think she is an attractive person.

Although Jessica has had a loyal group of friends since kindergarten, she has convinced herself that the only reason they are still friends with her is because they are too nice to tell her that they don't like her anymore. She is certain that no one wants to be friends with a "fat girl" and is waiting for the day her friends tell her she is no longer welcome to hang out with them. Any criticism she hears from them as well as others she interprets as an indirect criticism of her weight.

Jessica has developed an interest in dating boys her age but is terrified of expressing interest in anyone out of fear that they will make fun of her. She has heard others make fun of girls who are fatter than she. One of Jessica's male acquaintances did tell her that she is pretty but that she might not get any dates until she loses some weight, which further reinforced her idea that she is not really likeable because of the way she looks.

At her annual checkup before the school year began, her pediatrician talked with her about the importance of exercise and eating healthy. Jessica stated that she understood how important that was, that she did not often eat unhealthy foods like chips, cookies, or ice cream, and that she liked to go on long, 30–45-minute walks around her neighborhood most days of the week. Her pediatrician stated that she doubted Jessica had been doing those things and encouraged Jessica to tell her the truth, because if she really was eating healthy and exercising the way she said she was, she would not be overweight. Jessica left the appointment feeling dejected and disgusted with herself for not being a better, more attractive person.

She vowed to eat even healthier than she already was and to ramp up her exercise. She decided to cut out all sources of high-sugar and high-fat foods and began limiting the amount of food she would eat, no matter how healthy the food was, until she was eating around 1,000 calories a day. She also took up jogging. So instead of her leisurely walks through her neighborhood, she worked her way up to jogging up to five miles a day. She was hungry most of the time but was seeing some weight loss. Her friends and peers noticed and often complimented her on how she looked and encouraged her to "keep it up." She was able to sustain this regimen for several weeks before she "caved in" and gorged herself on all the junk food she could find in her house until she was so full she felt like she might throw up without trying. During her binge eating episode she felt a sense of relief and elation; however, immediately following the binge she felt disgusted with herself and started hitting herself in the stomach. Although she did not have another binge episode like that, she found that she was back to her previous eating habits— eating mostly healthy foods but more calories than she had been eating while dieting. It did not take long for her clothes to feel tighter and for her to need to buy clothes one size larger. She weighed herself and realized that she had gained the weight she had lost plus an additional five pounds.

After her weight gain, her friends and family were kind to her but typically asked things like "What happened? You were doing so well!" Despite their best intentions, questions and comments such as these only fueled her ever-growing feeling that she was a failure, a terrible person, and didn't deserve to feel good about herself. She thought about resuming the regimen that had resulted in weight loss but couldn't face feeling hungry all of the time. This led her to feel even worse about herself, and slowly she began eating "junk food" to help herself feel better.

Analysis

Jessica's experience of ultimately gaining weight plus more as a result of calorie restriction and increased exercise is typical of nearly all dieters. The research routinely shows that most people who go on some kind of diet do not maintain the weight loss over the long term. Additionally, some research has concluded that the most likely long-term outcome of any diet plan is weight gain, not weight loss.

What seems most unfortunate about Jessica's experience is that she was engaged in a healthy lifestyle prior to trying to lose weight. She was eating mostly healthy foods, not restricting her caloric intake, and was exercising regularly by doing something she enjoyed. What triggered her weight-loss attempt was a combination of low self-confidence and low self-esteem, overhearing others' comments about peers who were larger than she, her male friend's comment about needing to lose weight if she wanted to have a boyfriend, and her pediatrician's disbelief that she could be overweight while engaged in healthy behaviors.

Girls are more likely to experience the negative effects of being over-weight or obese, and while she did not appear to be experiencing bullying, she heard just enough from her peers and others to confirm for her that she was not worthy of friends or someone to date as long as she weighed as much as she did. Unfortunately, her attempts at weight loss, though common enough, resulted in what would be predicted from an attempt to lose weight via calorie restriction and an increase in exercise. She was unable to sustain such a restrictive diet and ended up in a binge eating episode. Although one episode does not equal an eating disorder, should Jessica continue a pattern of calorie restriction and binge eating, she may put herself at risk for developing an eating disorder. Additionally, her experience of feeling uncomfortably full to the point that she felt as if she might throw up may lead her to self-induce vomiting to relieve the discomfort should she engage in future binge eating episodes.

CASE 2: ROGER

Roger is a 17-year-old athlete who is a senior in high school. He has played football most of his life, starting with Pop Warner (i.e., pee wee) football at the age of five. Over the years he has developed his skills in a variety of positions on both the defensive and offensive side of the ball; however, it became clear to him and his coaches early on that he was very good as an offensive lineman as he had good reflexes and good ability to stand his ground. Although his coaches never explicitly told Roger to put on weight, he often overheard various coaches talk about "the bigger the better" when it came to playing offensive line and about how weight and strength combined with short bursts of speed from side to side and good hands for tackling made for the "perfect O-lineman."

Over the years, Roger put a lot of energy into making himself into the perfect player for this position. He was often one of the first in and last out when it came to practice days that involved weight training. He also increased his caloric intake, not only because he was hungrier, having built more muscle mass and burned a lot of energy during his workouts, but because he wanted to build even more muscle. Unfortunately, he surpassed his caloric needs so much that his body started to store the excess energy as body fat. Initially, this served him well as the extra weight made it more difficult for his opponents to move him out of the way. As he continued to put on weight, he noticed that he was not as agile as he had been. His opponents still found it difficult to move him out of the way, but when he was faced with a defensive lineman who was faster than he was, he was unable to react as quickly and effectively as he had been able to prior to putting on additional weight.

In addition to the changes he experienced as a player, he occasionally overheard his peers, some of whom were on the team and many of whom were simply fellow classmates, talk about how fat he was now. At times he heard people making fun of his weight and imitating him as if he were unable to move his body around without great effort. Roger began to worry that his plan to become the best offensive lineman he could had backfired. He felt ostracized and disconnected from his peers and began to withdraw from some of the classmates he had considered to be friends.

He was conflicted about what to do, as he had been heavily recruited by top-level Division I college football teams, which seemed to happen only after he was able to get bigger. He was afraid, however, that they would no longer be interested or that they would ultimately cut him from the team once they saw how big he had gotten. This thought process led to a drop in overall mood and an increase in anxiety about what he should do. He was too embarrassed to talk with his coaches and didn't trust his teammates to take him seriously. Moreover, his parents seemed so excited that he was going to play Division I football that he didn't want to disappoint them by saying he might be too fat to play at that level. This led Roger to feel even more isolated and disconnected from those who were important to him and who might have been able to help him. As a result, he turned to food to soothe his low mood and feelings of anxiousness.

This led to a vicious cycle of his feeling even worse about himself because he was eating mostly junk food and eating even more than he had been before, putting on more weight, which led him to feel badly about himself and turn to food to soothe himself. At this point, he knew he had put on so much weight that he was finding it difficult to move his body around the way he wanted and needed to, primarily on the football field, and underclass teammates were starting to outperform him. His coaches noticed this too and told him to "get his act together" or he would not be a starter for the current season, which could jeopardize his chances of signing with a Division I collegiate team.

Analysis

Roger's status as an athlete, particularly in a sport and in a position (i.e., offensive lineman) that requires a larger-sized body to be effective, may put him at increased risk for struggling to maintain the weight expectations of the sport. Although he does not appear to have an eating disorder, it is possible that he may develop a cycle of binge eating behavior when he feels badly about himself or anxious about whether or not his collegiate football career will even happen. What seems to be exacerbating much of Roger's struggle is that he is not consulting with or confiding in anyone that he is struggling to live up to the expectations of the sport and of his coaches (both current and potential future coaches). He is, therefore, struggling to manage not only his weight but also his emotions on his own; however, he does not appear to have the tools to adequately handle either.

Ideally, someone close to him will notice that something seems amiss. They may notice his weight gain, but they may also notice his change in mood and his tendency to withdraw from others, which has been atypical of him. Unfortunately, his coaches did notice a decline in his performance but simply told him to figure it out rather than checking in with him to see if anything were wrong and to offer assistance. Roger would benefit greatly from talking with someone (e.g., counselor, school counselor, trusted friend, or adult) about his concerns and fears about his body and his football career. He would also likely benefit greatly from consulting with a registered dietician who specializes in working with athletes so he can learn how much food and what types of foods to consume, and when he should consume them in order to build the body strength and size he has been searching for without compromising his speed and agility.

CASE 3: DANA

Dana is an 18-year-old first-year college student who is nearing comple-
tion of her first year. She easily made friends and had comfortably settled
into a new routine, living in the dorms, going to classes, studying, and
hanging out with friends, and often stated to her family how much she
loved college. She began college slightly overweight but was never concerned about her weight as she was an active child and teenager who ate
a broad range of food. She also had the tendency to eat when she was
hungry and stop when she was full, only occasionally overeating on occa-
sions like Thanksgiving. She had heard about the "freshman 15" prior to
starting college and, therefore, expected to gain some weight. As the year
progressed, however, she found that she gained a significant amount of
weight within the first semester and continued to gain more during the
second semester. At a recent doctor's visit, her physician told that her she
was close to being categorized as obese and that she needed to lose weight
in order to be healthy. She inquired about how she was unhealthy, and her
physician told her that there were no signs yet that her health had been
compromised but that the weight gain she experienced, particularly if she
continued to gain weight, meant that it would "only be a matter of time"
before she developed something like diabetes or high blood pressure. Her
physician additionally stated that if Dana did not get a handle on things
now, she'd likely develop heart disease and could have a stroke at some
point in the future.

Dana was sufficiently scared by what her physician said. She did not
feel unwell prior to her appointment, but in the weeks that followed she
became hyperaware of any changes in how her body felt and wondered if
she were already showing signs of some of the diseases he mentioned. Her
friends became worried about her as she started to consistently ask them
about various physical symptoms, like a random pain somewhere in her
body, heart palpitations, and headaches, and wondered if they experienced stuff like that too. They tried to reassure her by saying that those
things were normal and not to worry about it, but Dana was becoming
consumed by worry about her body and her weight.

Dana drastically cut back on the amount and types of food she ate,
which meant that she was not eating what her friends ate, and she started
to avoid hanging out with them as there was inevitably junk food or pizza
involved in their get-togethers. She also started to exercise on her own. As
a full-time student, she had access to the school's fitness center and started
working out there daily. Her efforts "paid off" in the sense that she began
losing weight. Initially, her friends and acquaintances were encouraging of

her efforts and complimented her on how she looked. She was also aware of the attention she was getting from male classmates, some of whom talked with her for the first time since college started. She was invigorated by the praise and attention she received and more fully committed to her efforts. She cut back further on her caloric intake and cut out more types of food. She also decided she had time to work out twice every day during the week and three times on the weekend. She was committing so much time and effort to her eating and exercise behaviors that she stopped hanging out with her friends altogether, politely declined any inquiries she received from male classmates about going on a date, and skipped studying if she hadn't been able to get her exercise in earlier in the day.

Dana's weight loss became so dramatic that the manager of the fitness center pulled her aside one morning and inquired about whether or not she was okay. Dana was confused by this concern because she was certain that losing weight was a good thing and no cause for alarm. Rather, it should be an indicator of her health. The manager stated that he was concerned that she was "overdoing" her exercising and that others had expressed concern to him about the intensity and frequency of her workouts as well as her dramatic weight loss, which some indicated seemed "unhealthy." Dana became angry at the manager and told him to mind his own business. He let her know that in order to keep working out in the fitness center, she would need to have a note from her doctor saying she was cleared for working out. Dana left the center angry and went on a 10-mile run.

Analysis

Dana began her college career as a healthy, happy young woman. She gained more weight than she may have expected and was told by her physician that it was imperative that she lose weight as soon as possible as her weight gain put her at greater risk for serious medical problems, and he stated that one or more of these diseases were inevitable if she continued to gain weight. As a result, Dana became overly focused on her body and how it felt, seemingly convinced that her normal aches and pains were signs of a serious illness her physician had predicted. This experience further motivated her to lose weight by whatever means necessary.

Although it is not clear how much weight Dana lost, her behaviors and weight loss caught the attention of those around her, including those at the campus fitness center. Her frequency, intensity, and duration of workouts along with significant weight loss caused concern among fellow exercisers and led to her not being able to use the facility until her physician stated that she was healthy to continue exercising. It is also unclear whether or not Dana plans to seek medical clearance; however, her response to the interaction with the fitness center manager suggests that she may no longer workout there and will only engage in workouts on her own (e.g., going on a 10-mile run).

Her current exercise and eating behaviors, her noticeable weight loss, her change in demeanor, and her withdrawal from friends and schoolwork suggest that Dana may have developed a significant mental health issue. Although there is not enough data to identify a diagnosis, it is possible that Dana has developed anorexia nervosa and may have developed some form of anxiety or illness anxiety disorder (formally known as hypochondriasis).

CASE 4: SYLVIA

Sylvia is a 16-year-old high school student. She has been identified as obese since childhood and has been placed on numerous diet and exercise plans throughout her life to try to lose weight and get to a normal weight range according to the BMI. Both of her parents and her younger brother are overweight or obese, and Sylvia has memories of going on more than one "family" diet whereby everyone in the family participated in changing their eating and exercise habits.

Growing up, food was always out and available, particularly "junk food" such as chips, cookies, crackers, and so on. Her memories of growing up to this day include everyone in her family eating nearly all the time. Almost everyone would have a box or bag of food they'd be eating while watching TV, playing games, or whatever they would be doing in between mealtimes. Sylvia also learned that food has been a source of comfort. Growing up, whenever she or her brother got hurt or were upset for some reason, their parents would offer them cookies or ice cream in order to cheer them up and make them feel better. As a result, Sylvia continues to turn to food whenever she feels upset in some way. She is aware of initially feeling good and has a sense of satisfaction after eating, but as she continues to eat she "zones out" and feels "numb." After she finishes eating, usually when whatever she is eating has run out, her initial thought is to eat more food. When she realizes how much she has eaten, she becomes more aware of herself and her body. She feels disgusted with herself and mentally rips herself apart for having eating so much food, particularly since the food is also high calorie and often high in sugar content and/or high in fat. She vows to herself that she will not do this again but finds herself resuming the same behaviors whenever she feels badly.

Sylvia has tried talking with her parents about how bad she feels about herself, her weight, and her eating habits. Their response is typically to reassure her that "everything will be okay" and that she "is a beautiful girl just as she is." They also acknowledge her struggle and admit to having similar thoughts and feelings about themselves. It is at these times that her family declares that they will all begin watching what they eat and will start exercising. They all participate in gathering up and throwing away all the junk food in the house and agree that no one will bring junk food back into the house. They also agree to go on a family walk following dinner each night for as long as they can, with the goal of a 30-minute walk. Each member of the family is able to fully participate in the plan for the better part of a week. Then, at least one family member will skip the walk because they feel too tired that day but promises to resume again the next day, or because they had a particularly stressful day, they allow themselves a "treat" of some kind. This has typically led to a slippery slope for all family members. Some are able to "hold out" longer than others; however, usually by the end of two weeks, all family members are back to eating as they always have, junk food is back in the house in large quantities, and their walks have all but ceased.

Sylvia, determined to do things differently than her family always has, decided to change her eating and exercise habits on her own. She was initially successful in making changes that her family did not seem to notice; however, when they realized she wasn't eating as they did while watching television or that she was consistently going out for a walk in the evening, they started asking her questions about what she was doing. They were supportive by saying things like "Good for you," "I'm proud of you," or "Keep it up." However, after a few days she started to feel pressure from them, particularly her mom and dad, to eat as they did and to not go for walks. They often offered her snacks during times she was not eating (e.g., sitting in front of the TV or while working on her computer) and said things like "Are you sure you have to go for a walk now?" and "We'll miss you." Eventually, she felt that whatever benefit she was gaining by changing her behaviors was outweighed by her family's efforts to get her to act like them again.

Analysis

It is possible that Sylvia has the genetics that will make her body more likely to store fat and a metabolism that does not burn as many calories as others'. This is likely a factor for her body weight and size. Additionally, her family has a collective set of habits that are not terribly healthy. As a family, they seem to recognize that their eating and exercise habits are not ideal (though it is not clear whether they think this for health reasons or simply from the perspective of body weight and size), as evidenced by their efforts to eat differently and to engage in exercise. Moreover, there is no evidence that any of the members of the family have formal support (e.g., a counselor) for their efforts, which makes maintaining these new behaviors particularly difficult. This is likely why the new behaviors rarely last for more than one or two weeks.

It is often the case that eating junk food predominantly and in the way that this family seems to is an indicator that they are using food to cope with stress and unpleasant emotional experiences, though this is clear only with Sylvia. When one's primary or only coping mechanism is taken away for whatever reason, it is important to know what other coping mechanisms can be used instead and to have someone to help them through particularly difficult times when one's energy levels or willpower are low and they require an extraordinary amount of effort to continue with new coping behaviors (see Question 19 for more information about willpower). In Sylvia's case, she would also benefit from learning how to respectfully "push back" against her family when they are encouraging her to eat like them again and to not exercise. It is not clear that any of her family members are maliciously trying to sabotage her efforts; however, efforts that exert pressure on someone to resume "regular behaviors," no matter the intention, can be difficult to resist, particularly if one does not know what to say or how to react.

CASE 5: DREW

Drew is a 22-year-old male who has graduated from college and has begun his career in his first salaried position. Drew was fairly active in high school and throughout college; however, his job requires him to work long hours and sit most of the time at a desk, working on a computer. Since he started his new job a year ago, he has noticed that his weight has increased and his clothes no longer fit him. He continues to work out one or two days of the week, but his workouts tend to be much briefer than they used to be (i.e., 20 or 30 minutes rather than an hour or more) because he is too tired after working all day to put in more time than that at the gym. Drew has realized that being healthy requires more effort than it did when he was in high school and college but has been unable to figure out how to reprioritize his health. Drew was always overweight but felt healthy and energized as an adolescent and throughout college. Now his weight increase has put him close to the obese range of the BMI chart.

Some of his co-workers have teased him about his weight, commenting on his "beer belly" and mentioning that he looks "flabby" now. Although intended to be good-natured teasing, Drew has become more self-conscious about how he looks, particularly around his waist. This has been particularly distressing for Drew since the summer months are approaching when he would typically spend more time outdoors, including at the local beach, and wear clothes such as shorts, t-shirts, and a bathing suit, which reveal more of his body than colder-weather clothing. He usually gets together with his friends and never thought twice about wearing less clothing (i.e., summer clothes) or taking his shirt off if he got hot enough. Now, however, he is dreading this time of year and the accompanying invitations to do something outdoors with his friends.

Drew scheduled an appointment with his primary care provider to inquire about his overall health. His physician confirmed that he has put on weight but that his vitals and blood chemistry are all within the healthy range. His physician stated that he is, in fact, in good health and encouraged Drew to eat as healthy as possible but not to cut out his favorite foods; rather, limit them if they have a high fat or high sugar content. He also encouraged Drew to continue his workouts and to try to work out at least three days per week for 30 minutes a day doing something he enjoys. Drew's physician also encouraged him to get up from his desk and stand or walk around for a few minutes every hour since sitting for hours at a time is unhealthy even for those who exercise every day. Finally, he encouraged Drew to focus on engaging in healthy behaviors (i.e., eating reasonably and exercising reasonably) and trying not to focus on his weight. He added that he may very well lose some weight should he find time to exercise more and limit his consumption of less healthy foods but that the most important thing is to take care of his body, and his weight will be whatever it needs to be.

Drew tried to take this advice to heart; however, he couldn't stop thinking about all the weight he put on, how his co-workers and friends teased him about it, and how he wanted to look more attractive, which for him meant he needed to lose weight. Drew tried for several weeks to work out as he used to when he was in college, which meant he was getting up early to work out for at least an hour before his day began rather than waiting until the end of the day. He did some kind of intense cardio three days per week and lifted weights twice per week. On weekends he would go for a run for at least an hour, with the goal of running farther each time. Drew also cut out sweets, chips, and fried foods entirely. After a couple of weeks he had lost several pounds, which was noticeable to those who knew him. Some praised him for his efforts, while others teased him about "getting skinny." Drew was pleased with his efforts and his results but found that he was craving the foods he had eliminated from his diet and that he was finding it more and more difficult to get himself out of bed in the morning to exercise. After another week of his new routine, he started skipping some of his morning workouts and allowing himself to "indulge" in some of the foods he had not been allowing himself to eat. Shortly thereafter, Drew was no longer working out at all and was eating whatever food he wanted but in larger quantities than he had been before. It was not long before his weight started to increase.

Analysis

Drew seems to have experienced what a lot of people do as the summer months approach. He became more concerned about how he would look in summer clothing, which tends to be more revealing than clothes worn during other months of the year. The comments and teasing from his co-workers and friends did nothing to help Drew keep his body weight and size in perspective. Drew sought the advice of his primary care physician and to see whether or not he was medically unhealthy due to his weight gain. Although it is not clear, it is likely that his physician has taken the Health at Every Size® perspective as evidenced by encouraging Drew to focus on engaging in healthy behaviors rather than focusing exclusively on his weight. Despite this advice, Drew remained focused on his weight and did what many people do, which was to start a new diet and workout regimen by restricting the quantity and types of food he ate and engaging in increased exercise. Although this is not necessarily a bad approach, it is typically unsustainable for the majority of people (i.e., over 95 percent cannot sustain such a regimen). Drew would be well served to start with his physician's recommendations to engage in exercise that he enjoys for a shorter amount of time and fewer days of the week, and to allow himself to eat all of the foods he would like and limit (but not exclude) foods that are high in fat and high in sugar. It may be possible from that point forward to add more days or time to his exercise routine if he has the time and energy given his work schedule. He may also find that by eating primarily healthy foods, but still having some less healthy foods, and exercising, his body shape may change in a way that he likes but that may not show much of a change on the scale.

Glossary

Adipose tissue: Adipose tissue is the technical term used for body fat.

Adiposity: Adiposity refers to being overweight or obese.

Adiposity rebound: After a period of rapid increase in BMI, which usually peaks around 9–12 months of age, a child's BMI will start to decline. The point at which a child's BMI reaches its lowest point (i.e., maximal leanness or minimal BMI) is referred to as adiposity rebound. The average age of adiposity rebound is between ages five and six.

Anorexia nervosa: Anorexia nervosa is an eating disorder characterized by loss of a significant amount of body weight by restricting food intake, which ultimately leads to a very low body weight, a fear of gaining weight or being fat regardless of body size, and the inability to accurately perceive one's body size.

Anti-fat bias: Anti-fat bias reflects a negative attitude toward individuals who have fat bodies (usually overweight or obese) that can lead to a negative attitude toward the person and not just their body (e.g., that they are lazy or stupid). The opposite of this is the pro-thin bias.

Bariatric surgery: Bariatric surgery is the technical term for weight-loss surgery that involves changing the digestive tract for the purpose of weight loss and prevention of subsequent weight gain.

Behavior management: In the context of obesity, behavior management refers to techniques, which can be self-taught or taught to someone by a counselor or psychotherapist, designed to help individuals control their weight. Often behavior management involves helping individuals identify and manage barriers preventing them from losing weight and learning new thoughts and behaviors that promote weight loss and prevent weight gain.

Binge eating: This is a term used in the context of a mental health diagnosis, particularly eating disorders, and refers to eating a large quantity of food in a relatively short period of time compared to what is typically consumed under similar circumstances. Binge eating episodes are part of binge eating disorder and bulimia nervosa.

Binge eating disorder: Binge eating disorder is a mental health diagnosis that involves engaging in binge eating episodes and feeling as if the person cannot stop binge eating. The disorder is typically accompanied by eating quickly, feeling excessively full, eating a lot even when not hungry, feeling embarrassed by how much one has eaten, and feeling disgusted with oneself or guilty after a binge.

BMI report cards: Used in school settings, BMI report cards are sent home with the student that indicate the child's height, weight, and BMI. The report may include recommendations for the student and family based on the child's BMI. Not all schools use BMI report cards, and some that have used them have discontinued using them due to public backlash and concern for harm.

Body dissatisfaction: Body dissatisfaction refers to negative thoughts and feelings one has about one's body. It can occur in men and women at any body weight, shape, or size.

Body mass index (BMI): BMI is a mathematical formula that divides a person's weight by their height (squared). The equation was developed in the mid 1800s for the purpose of studying populations and to determine the "average man." It is currently used by most primary care providers as an indicator of one's overall health.

Body positivity: Body positivity refers to the attitude of accepting and appreciating all shapes and sizes of the human body, including one's own.

Bulimia nervosa: Bulimia nervosa is a mental health diagnosis that involves binge eating episodes and engaging in some type of compensatory behavior in order to get rid of the calories consumed during a binge.

Centers for Disease Control and Prevention (CDC): The CDC is an agency of the U.S. federal government tasked with intervention and prevention efforts related to public health.

Circadian rhythm: A circadian rhythm is any biological process that operates based on a 24-hour cycle.

Cognitive-behavioral therapy (CBT): CBT is a form of counseling that addresses thought patterns in order to change unwanted and/or harmful patterns of behavior.

Compensatory behaviors: This is a term used in the context of the eating disorder bulimia nervosa to refer to behaviors designed to prevent weight gain. These behaviors include self-induced vomiting, the use of laxatives or diuretics or other medications that may result in weight loss, fasting, or excessive exercise.

Eating disorders: Eating disorders are a class of mental health disorders now listed and described under the category of Feeding and Eating Disorders in the *Diagnostic and Statistical Manual of Mental Disorders-5* (DSM-5). Eating disorders include anorexia nervosa, bulimia nervosa, and binge eating disorder, all of which are characterized by abnormal eating behaviors.

Excessive exercise: This is a term that has multiple definitions and usually refers to exercise that is more than is necessary to maintain one's health and well-being, that may interfere with one's health and well-being, and that may be reflected in feelings of guilt or irritability when the individual is not able to engage in exercise.

Fight or flight: This term refers to the physiological arousal of the sympathetic nervous system (a branch of the autonomic nervous system) and is characterized by physiological changes such as an increase in heart rate, blood pressure, and skin temperature. The fight or flight response is activated when there is a perceived threat or attack.

Food desert: This is a term used to describe a geographical area in which affordable and healthy foods (e.g., fresh fruits and vegetables) are difficult to buy either because they are unaffordable or because the nearest location to get such food is too far away.

Food insecurity: This is a term used to describe situations in which access to enough affordable and healthy foods (e.g., fresh fruits and vegetables) is not reliable.

Food security: Food security refers to the condition that all people at all times have easy and reliable access to affordable and healthy foods (e.g., fresh fruits and vegetables) that meet one's dietary needs and preferences in support of a healthy life.

"Freshman 15": This is a term used to refer to the weight gain that often occurs among first-year college students who are often not as active as they had been in high school and are also likely eating less healthy food as they have more access to a wider variety of food choices and may be more likely to consume less healthy food overall.

Health at Every Size®: This is an approach adopted by those who endorse the idea that one's health status is a result of healthy or unhealthy behaviors rather than body size. Thus, they suggest that our emphasis should be on encouraging people to engage in healthy eating habits and healthy exercise habits rather than weight loss. This approach is based on the book *Health at Every Size: The Surprising Truth about Your Weight* by Linda Bacon.

Hypochondriasis: See illness anxiety disorder.

Illness anxiety disorder: Formerly known as hypochondriasis, this psychiatric disorder involves someone who is excessively worried about being seriously ill or becoming seriously ill. Often there are no physical symptoms of illness, or minor symptoms are viewed by the individual as a sign of a serious illness.

Metabolic syndrome: Metabolic syndrome refers to a set of physiological factors that contribute to diseases such as heart disease, diabetes, and stroke. Having at least three of the five factors known to contribute to these diseases warrants a diagnosis of metabolic syndrome. The five factors are excess abdominal fat (i.e., a large waistline), high triglycerides, low HDL cholesterol, high blood pressure, and high fasting blood sugar.

Metabolism: This includes all the biochemical processes that occur within the body in order to sustain the life of the body.

Muscular-ideal: This is the term used to describe the ideal male body in western cultures. It is characterized by well-defined muscles and low body fat.

National Organization for Women (NOW): NOW was established in 1966 with the mission of opposing sex discrimination and enacting equality for all women.

Obesity: Obesity refers to the state of one's body as excessively overweight or fat. When measured using BMI, obesity in adults occurs when one's BMI is 30.0 or higher. For children and adolescents, obesity occurs when one's BMI is at or above the 95th percentile for someone of the same age and sex.

Overweight: Overweight refers to the state of one's body that is above a weight that is considered "normal" or "desirable." When measured using BMI, overweight in adults is defined as a BMI that is at least 25.0 but less than 30.0. For children and adolescents, overweight is defined as a BMI that is above the 85th percentile but less than the 95th percentile compared to those of the same age and sex.

Pro-thin bias: Pro-thin bias reflects a positive attitude toward individuals who have thin bodies that can lead to a positive attitude toward the person and not just their body (e.g., that they are smart, are motivated, have high self-control). The opposite of this is the anti-fat bias.

Purging behavior: In the context of eating disorders, purging behavior refers to any behavior designed to get rid of food. The most common method of purging is self-induced vomiting.

Registered dietitian: Registered dietitians are experts in food and nutrition who have at least a bachelor's degree, who have practiced under supervision in the context of an accredited program, and who have passed a national examination. Typically, registered dietitians are licensed by the state in which they practice.

Sarcopenia: This is the natural loss of muscle tissue associated with aging.

Set-point: With regard to weight, set-point refers to a range of body weight at which an individual's body will function at its best.

Size acceptance: Also referred to as "fat acceptance," size acceptance is a socially based grassroots movement with the mission of changing anti-fat bias and negative social attitudes with regard to weight, specifically overweight and obesity.

Socioeconomic status (SES): SES refers to the social standing (i.e., class) of a person or a group of people typically based on level of education, income, and type of occupation.

Stress hormones: These are the hormones in the body that are released when the body and/or the person is under stress. Stress hormones include cortisol, adrenaline, and norepinephrine. Cortisol is often referred to as "the stress hormone," and chronically high levels of cortisol can lead to things such as immune system suppression, increase in blood pressure, and increase in blood sugar levels.

Thin-ideal: This is the ideal body type for females in western cultures that is characterized by a thin and curvy but lean body with low body fat.

Weight cycling: See yo-yo dieting.

Weight-loss medications: These are medications prescribed specifically for weight loss. Some medications suppress one's feeling of hunger or make one feel full faster, whereas others may make it more difficult for one's body to absorb and store fat.

Weight-loss surgery: Also known as bariatric surgery, weight-loss surgery refers to a set of surgical procedures that change the digestive system in order to promote weight loss and prevent weight gain.

Yo-yo dieting: Also known as weight cycling, the term refers to a pattern of repeatedly losing then gaining weight and can result in things such as high blood pressure, high cholesterol, diabetes, heart disease, and some forms of cancer.

Directory of Resources

BOOKS

Bacon, L. (2008). *Health at Every Size: The Surprising Truth about Your Weight*. Dallas, TX: BenBella Books, Inc.

Brownell, K. D., and B. T. Walsh. (2017). *Eating Disorders and Obesity: A Comprehensive Handbook (3rd Ed.)*. New York: Guilford Press.

Fung, J., and T. Noakes. (2016). *The Obesity Code: Unlocking the Secrets of Weight Loss*. Vancouver, Canada: Greystone Books.

Gaesser, G. A. (2002). *Big Fat Lies: The Truth about Your Weight and Your Health*. Carlsbad, CA: Gürze Books.

Selby, C. L. B. (2017). *The Body Size and Health Debate*. Santa Barbara, CA: Greenwood.

ORGANIZATIONS

American Medical Association (AMA)

https://www.ama-assn.org/

Founded in 1847, the AMA is the largest association of medical doctors and medical students in the United States. The purpose of the association is to promote scientific efforts, establish standards for medical education, establish medical ethics, and find ways to improve public health.

Association for Size Diversity and Health (ASDAH)

https://www.sizediversityandhealth.org/index.asp

ASDAH is a nonprofit organization focused on the tenets of the Health at Every Size® approach to wellness. Their focus is on helping to prevent size discrimination, to ensure that those who are overweight or obese have equal access to services, healthcare, and other resources, and to support their overall wellbeing.

The Campaign to End Obesity

http://www.obesitycampaign.org/

This organization, headquartered in Washington, D.C., works to "fill the gap" in efforts to "reverse" the obesity epidemic by providing information and consultation to stakeholders in the treatment and prevention of obesity.

Centers for Disease Control and Prevention (CDC)

https://www.cdc.gov/

The CDC is an agency of the federal government housed under the U.S. Department of Health and Human Services. The mission of the CDC is the protection of the citizens of the United States from threats to their health, safety, and security. Their primary focus is on diseases that may have developed in country or abroad but that may make their way to the United States.

Food and Drug Administration (FDA)

https://www.fda.gov/

Part of the Department of Health and Human Services, the FDA is a governmental agency of the United States charged with protecting public health by regulating and ensuring the safety of things such as prescription medications, medical devices, and the food supply.

National Heart, Lung, and Blood Institute (NHLBI)

https://www.nhlbi.nih.gov/

Part of the U.S. Department of Health and Human Services, the NHLBI conducts research on the prevention, diagnosis, and treatment of diseases of the heart, lungs, and blood. They also fund outside research and clinical trials related to their focus.

Obesity Action Coalition (OAC)

https://www.obesityaction.org/
The OAC is a nonprofit organization focused on the "disease of obesity," providing assistance to individuals and their families. They focus on obesity prevention and treatment and provide education related to fighting weight-based prejudice and discrimination and about how weight impacts health.

The Obesity Society

https://www.obesity.org/
This organization was founded in 1982 for professionals focused on the science, treatment, and prevention of obesity.

World Health Organization (WHO)

http://www.who.int/
The WHO was established on April 7, 1948, the day each year that is celebrated as World Health Day. The WHO is headquartered in Switzerland and has personnel in 150 countries worldwide. The WHO works within the system of the United Nations to ensure the health and well-being of all human beings across the globe.

World Obesity Federation

https://www.worldobesity.org/
A professional organization with members from scientific, medical, and research backgrounds. They aim to lead worldwide efforts to reduce, prevent, and treat obesity.

WEBSITES

American Diabetes Association—The obesity paradox

http://www.diabetes.org/research-and-practice/we-are-research-leaders/recent-advances/archive/the-obesity-paradox.html

American Heart Association

http://www.heart.org/HEARTORG/HealthyLiving/WeightManage-
ment/Obesity/Obesity-Information_UCM_307908_Article.jsp

American Medical Association—Report of the Council on Science and Public Health

https://www.ama-assn.org/sites/default/files/media-browser/public/
about-ama/councils/Council%20Reports/council-on-science-pub-
lic-health/a13csaph3.pdf

American Medical Association—Addressing Childhood Obesity

https://www.ama-assn.org/sites/default/files/media-browser/spe-
cialty%20group/arc/addressing-childhood-obesity-issue-brief.pdf

American Psychological Association

http://www.apa.org/topics/obesity/index.aspx

HealthyChildren.Org

https://www.healthychildren.org/English/health-issues/conditions/obe-
sity/Pages/default.aspx

KidsHealth

https://kidshealth.org/en/parents/overweight-obesity.html

Nutrition.gov

https://www.nutrition.gov/subject/nutrition-and-health-issues/
overweight-and-obesity

The State of Obesity

https://stateofobesity.org/

STOP Obesity Alliance

http://stopobesityalliance.org/

Index

About the Author

Christine L. B. Selby is a licensed psychologist, sport psychologist, and eating disorder specialist. She is also an associate professor of psychology at Husson University and maintains a part-time private practice with Selby Psychological Services, PLLC. She is a Certified Eating Disorder Specialist with the International Association of Eating Disorders Professionals (iaedp™) and was the co-founder (2008) and co-chair (2008–2014) of the Eating Disorders Special Interest Group of the Association for Applied Sport Psychology. Christine has published articles and book chapters in the area of eating disorders in athletes. She has also presented locally and nationally on eating disorders and related topics at professional conferences, and to allied professionals who work directly with those dealing with eating disorders and related concerns. Christine is the author of *Chilling Out: The Psychology of Relaxation*, *The Body Size and Health Debate*, and *The Psychology of Eating Disorders*.